GROW YOUR MIND, SHRINK YOUR WAIST

DEDICATIONS

I dedicate this book to my wife, Samantha,

and my precious daughter, Rosabelle.

This book is also dedicated to those who feel stagnant.

If you've plateaued, hit a wall, or just aren't seeing progress,

I know this book can change your life.

It was made with you in mind.

Contents

PART I: ACTION

PART II: LEARN

PART III: PURPOSE

INTRODUCTION

*T*he fitness industry can be extremely intimidating and confusing to outsiders. People jump from one fad to the next and wonder why they don't get any lasting results. Have you ever lost weight and seen some success only to have your progress come crashing down? Have you lost focus and ended up heavier or in more pain than you were when you started? Have you used the phrase "self-sabotage" to describe your weight-loss attempts?

There is a blueprint available that will show you what you'll need to see permanent results on your fitness journey. *Grow Your Mind, Shrink Your Waist* takes you through all the major steps that you'll go through on your adventure to a healthier you. We'll go over the major pitfalls and the ways to get around them. In this book, I won't teach you how to exercise or diet; I'll teach you how to structure your life, so those pieces will find their way in naturally.

As a regular guy, I was tired, out of shape, and unmotivated. When I made a career change to fitness and started applying the principles in this book, my life changed. I lost over 30 pounds and started living a fuller life. I have learned from some of the most knowledgeable fitness professionals in the industry, as well as other experts outside of fitness.

I have helped hundreds of people apply these principles to their lives and watched as their health, attitude, and physique transformed. I want to connect deeply with you. I want to engage the artistic right side of your brain with a story and allow your logical left side to absorb the information and analysis of that story.

Grow Your Mind, Shrink Your Waist has two parts to it. The first part is a story portion, where you can see the themes of the book lived out and modeled for you. The second part of the book breaks down the lessons and presents a practical approach to using what you absorbed through the story.

I could have written a book about how to grow your mind using only facts, research, and a few poignant anecdotes. I have chosen to add a story in addition to that because that is how we, as humans, think and connect. Story connects to the deepest part of our being, and we can remember a good story much longer than we can remember a good statistic.

Emotion drives action. If all it took to succeed was a checklist of what to do, you'd already have your results and wouldn't still be searching for the answer. It takes facts and emotional engagement to make changes; I know you'll find both in the pages ahead.

Let's hear from my friend and client, Cindy:

"I could hardly walk up a flight of stairs without becoming short of breath. I was tired and felt I was losing my edge at work. I tend to eat in response to stress. Although it was hard for me to admit, I needed help."

This is what Cindy said after following our program:

"I am amazed how much improvement I have seen in my strength, endurance, and aerobic capacity. I have lost 70 pounds in nine months and have not felt hungry or deprived. I am still surprised at how easy the weight loss has been. I have more energy than I have had in many years. I sleep better. I feel sharper. I walked up four flights of stairs at work the other day while carrying on a conversation — and did not think twice about it!

"I am doing things I only dreamed of doing last fall. I completed a 5K race (okay, I mostly walked) and have signed up for a paddleboard course. It's really fun to see someone I have not seen in a while. I have changed so much that sometimes, they don't recognize me."

Cindy has maintained this weight since September of 2016. That's a full two years of maintenance at the time of this writing. She has improved and grown in so many ways.

GROW YOUR MIND SHRINK YOUR WAIST

I guarantee my results. If you act on and apply the principles in this book, you will achieve your fitness and health goals. If you're after weight loss, it will become permanent weight loss. If you're building muscle, you'll grow it and look the best you ever have. I promise that these principles will take you where you want to go. Bear in mind that your results are only as permanent as the changes you're willing to stick with. If you're looking for a quick fix, a one-week detox, or a 21-day "shred-it" plan, you're in the wrong place.

Don't be the person who flounders year after year in a constant state of yo-yo dieting. Be the kind of person who breaks free from the vicious cycle of weight loss and gain. Be the kind of person other people look at and say, "You look great; what have you been doing?!" Be the kind of person who takes the necessary action and does it immediately.

The principles you're about to read will catapult you into the body and life of your dreams. All you need to do to unlock your potential is keep reading. Each chapter will follow the gripping story of a person who is not so different from you. Her circumstances are extraordinary, but the inner turmoil she experiences is all too common. She represents many of the clients I have trained over the years. I've incorporated many of their stories into her character. As our heroine follows the path of transformation, we'll recap the lesson at the end of each part. Let the story illuminate the path to a healthier, slimmer, and stronger you.

For those looking to get a head start, go to www.GrowYourMindBook.com to get the free 10 Day Jumpstart Course I've designed specifically to apply the concepts in this book in as short a time frame as possible.

Author's note: This book was designed to be read in multiple ways. If you're here for the experience as intended, turn the page and read on. If you want to immerse yourself in the story first, read the story portion of each part. If you're after the CliffsNotes version of the book, skip to the lesson and action points at the end of each part. However you choose your adventure, I know you'll get what you came for.

PROLOGUE

The world Kathy lives in is not so different from our own. Just below the surface of her modern world, however, lies magic. It has gone unnoticed for centuries. Most people don't believe it exists. However, there are still a few who believe. They know that a reckoning is coming, that the world has strayed too far.

Trolls are making a reemergence to teach the world a forgotten truth. They have survived in folklore as mythical creatures out to deceive and do harm to others. They existed to bring others down. Their civilization – if it can be called that – never amounted to much. They lived in caves and didn't leave any lasting impact, other than a legacy of negativity and a number of myths and stories used to teach lessons to children.

In Kathy's world, a curse has fallen upon the Earth, turning people into the trolls that they've so effectively imitated. Their shape is transformed, and their attitudes shift into permanent negativity. They are now the living embodiment of the worst traits of humanity.

People have never been more divided, isolated, or negative. The self-serving and selfish nature of society has turned people into monsters. They tweet, bully, and terrorize each other on a daily basis. Words have been used for millennia to build and create.

They are now being used on a massive scale to ruthlessly cut people down.

Kathy doesn't realize it, but the world is on the brink of changing for the worse. She is a good person with untapped potential, but she would not call herself a hero. In order to save the world and bring her husband back to her, she will need to adjust her mindset, change her body, and grow as a person.

PART I

ACTION

CHAPTER 1
Sick, Tired, and Ready for Change

The stale office air was especially dry this time of year. Kathy's ficus had seen better days. With the heat kicking on every few minutes to combat the sub-freezing temperatures outside, it sat on the corner of her desk, looking lonely and dejected as it withered. Kathy got up from her desk and strolled over to the water cooler.

A boisterous conversation conveniently broke up as she arrived.

"See you there?" Phil asked.

"I wouldn't miss it!" Sharon replied.

They were referring to trivia night at the local pub. Many of her coworkers attended, but Kathy had never been invited.

As she filled a cup of water for her parched plant, she noticed Ted's door opening. Ted was a tall man, probably six-foot-two. He was loud, had an aggressive handshake, and looked dapper in his tailored pants and designer shirts. "Management material" had been the phrase bandied about since he'd been hired eighteen months ago.

Despite her several years of seniority and experience, Kathy had been passed over for a promotion so that Ted could have his chance. And he was bound and determined to make the most of it.

Ted's long strides brought him to the water cooler in moments.

"Kathy," Ted said, his gaze fixed on her as she instinctively thought about running away. "Have you got all your ducks in a row on the Compact Solutions deal? I need you to send that marketing material out as soon as you get the chance. We've got to get these companies to buy-in if there's any hope of moving the needle on this quarter's goals. We're on a burning platform here, and Tom won't be happy if we're not making these conversions."

The speed and rapidity of his business jargon was another one of the subtly annoying things about Ted. It was like he only used words found in *Business Insider* and obscure marketing blogs. Letting her momentary irritation fade, Kathy refocused on his question and allusion to Tom, the unhappy CEO.

PART I: ACTION

"I have all the paperwork ready. I'm just waiting on Teresa to finish up the graphics," Kathy replied.

"Just make sure it's out by day's end. We don't want to miss our window of opportunity," Ted said as he pivoted and strode off to the next task on his planner.

Kathy took a long gulp of water and crushed the small paper cup in her hands. Five o'clock couldn't come soon enough.

After a slew of emails and time-wasting conversations, Kathy was able to get the materials sent out before day's end, as requested. As she started her car and left the office, she remembered that she'd never watered her plant. Tomorrow, she'd get another chance.

She pulled out into rush-hour traffic and ponderously made her way to the local grocery store.

Kathy grabbed the nearest cart and began filling it with what she guessed was what she needed. She had a written list but had left it on the kitchen counter. As Kathy mindlessly strolled through each aisle, she thought about work. The production company she worked for was one of the biggest in the area. It employed over 600 people in the factory and offices combined. She loved some of her coworkers; they were nice and genuine people. But it stressed her out just thinking about having Ted as her boss.

GROW YOUR MIND SHRINK YOUR WAIST

With a loaded shopping cart, Kathy stood in the checkout line. The magazines there always made her uncomfortable. Their messages screamed: *"Reinvigorate your sex life! EASY weight loss! Toned and skinny with this ONE NEW TRICK!"* All the marketing messages spoke to her needs, but she knew better than to go looking in the pages of a beauty magazine for real advice. What she needed was more discipline and a little bit of extra time. The weight would come off. She'd definitely gained since the last time she tried to lose weight, but that didn't matter.

The person in front of Kathy paid and left. The teenager at the register began scanning each of Kathy's items and placing them in the bags.

"Hello! Thank you for shopping at Food Paradise. Did you find everything okay?" the young man said, his voice clearly still in transition to adulthood.

"Yes, found everything just fine," Kathy replied. She noted his nametag: Skylar.

Beep. Beep. Skylar scanned two half-gallons of ice cream: Fudgsicle Delicious and Caramel Macchiato.

"Did you mean to get both of these?" he asked. "They aren't on sale anymore. Do you still want two?"

PART I: ACTION

Kathy turned crimson. "Two is just fine, thank you," she said through pursed lips. Kathy was sure she had never been more embarrassed than in that moment. Even a teenage boy was judging her choices. Kathy quickly paid and left the store. Her insides quaked with silent rage, embarrassment, and despair.

Kathy arrived home tired. The day had certainly not been a good one, and it was only Tuesday. As she unloaded her bags and put away the groceries, she noticed the list sitting on the counter. Milk and chicken were on the list, but she hadn't bought them.

Great, looks like I know where I'll be tomorrow.

She unpacked a bag of fresh spinach to put into the crisper and found last week's bag, unused and soggy. As she opened up the pantry, she saw duplicates of most of the canned goods she had purchased.

Frustrated, Kathy finished unpacking and putting everything away. When the thought of dinner and housework came into her head, she resigned herself to the couch and began thinking of easier options. Takeout came to mind.

Maybe that new Asian fusion restaurant that had just opened up…

Kathy's reverie was broken when Bill opened the back door and began stomping his feet to rid them of snow. Based on the volume and pace of his stomping, Kathy sensed that Bill was not in the best of moods.

"What's for dinner?" Bill bellowed from the kitchen.

Just once in our thirty years of marriage, could he ask me a different question when he gets home?

She could hear the refrigerator door open and close, followed by the cupboards.

"How about that new Asian fusion restaurant?" Kathy hollered back from the comfort of the living room.

Kathy heard a grunt and more shuffling around in the kitchen, which told her all she needed to know. No Asian food tonight. Kathy let out a sigh. As she mentally flipped through her rolodex of restaurants, she glanced downward. Slouched on the plush cushions of the couch, her "pooch" – as she called it – was on full display.

I need to get back to the gym.

Bill strolled into the living room with a beer and a bag of chips. He flopped into a chair and flipped on the television.

"You're going to spoil your dinner," Kathy said.

PART I: ACTION

"What dinner?" Bill said as he crunched loudly on his chips.

Touché.

Looked like it was a wine and ice cream kind of night. Quietly frustrated, Kathy vowed that tomorrow would be different. She left the comfy confines of the couch and headed into the kitchen.

Kathy poured a glass of red wine; a delicious, locally-grown vintage with a dryness that Kathy loved. She noticed that Bill had brought in the mail. On the counter were a few bills and some junk mail. Kathy quickly leafed through them. One piece caught her eye. It was for a local gym. The owner was a small-town celebrity. Across one side of the postcard, in bold letters, read: **"It's time to take care of you… and we're here to help!"** Kathy gave it a second glance, then threw it in the recycling bin.

When she returned to her post in the living room, Kathy could hear Bill grumbling about the game. He turned to her and gave her a loving glance.

"Hey, honey, sorry I've been a bear lately," Bill said. "I feel like these rotating hours are slowly killing me."

"Thanks, honey," Kathy replied.

He shot her another loving smile as she settled into reading the latest issue of *O, The Oprah Magazine*. Kathy smiled back with all the warmth that came with 25 years of a mostly happy marriage. Within twenty minutes, Bill was snoring soundly. Kathy looked at him and couldn't help thinking about their two children, Jacob and Hannah.

They were both off at school now. Jacob was graduating soon. He looked just like his father, from his build to his hair. He even had the independent streak to match.

Hannah was in her second year of school and was struggling with her course load. She had chosen the same school as Jacob and had pledged a sorority her first semester.

Kathy was worried about the choices they were making. They only talked to her once in awhile, but Kathy could see based on their social media posts that school wasn't all academics for them.

I miss our kids.

Kathy's gaze returned to Bill. Things were stagnant now. It was a new normal in the house. Less excitement and activity. They had both settled into the routines of work and relaxation. Their marriage was missing something, though Kathy couldn't place a finger on what.

PART I: ACTION

Kathy's spoon hit the bottom of the ice cream container – her cue to put it away. As Kathy threw out the accumulated garbage from the day, she could hear Bill rise from his chair.

By the time Kathy arrived in the bedroom, Bill's snores were hitting their crescendo. She slumped into bed, ready for the day to be over. It was difficult to find the first whispers of sleep, so Kathy reflected on her day. Her boss came to mind.

I wish he'd brush his teeth during the day. Would it be rude if I offered him some gum?

Kathy started thinking about her time on the couch. How lazy and empty she felt.

Is this what the rest of my fifties are going to be like?

That piece of junk mail came back to mind. Kathy hopped out of bed and fished the card out of the recycling bin. She placed it gingerly on the counter next to her keys. Kathy crept into the bedroom and back under the warmth of the sheets.

The gym. That's what she needed. She needed to get back into a routine. It felt like she had lost the same few pounds over and over again for as long as she could remember. Up, down. Up, down. They just kept coming back. Each time the pounds returned, they moved back in with all their baggage – both in the physical and metaphorical sense. Like a cruel joke, her excess fat continued to taunt her.

With that last thought, Kathy drifted off to sleep.

CHAPTER 2
Change Strikes

*T*he bedroom was dark, with a hint of light peeking through the shades.

Why hadn't the alarm gone off?

Kathy glanced over to see it blinking next to her. 2:33 AM strobed silently over and over.

So that means two-and-a-half hours ago, the power went out. Great.

Bill was an early riser and must not have noticed the clock blinking.

Kathy sprang out of bed to check the time on her phone. 7:45 AM. She was going to be late.

As Kathy zipped through her morning routine, she found a handwritten note on the counter. Quickly stuffing it into her pocket, she thought little else of Bill in her mad dash out the door. She grabbed her keys and the postcard.

GROW YOUR MIND SHRINK YOUR WAIST

Today, I'm making a call, Kathy vowed.

At 8:25 AM, Kathy opened her front door and pushed the button on her key fob to unlock the car. Kathy opened the door, sat down, and turned the ignition. The car started up quietly, and Kathy quickly got settled in her seat. As she looked up from her seatbelt, she knew something was terribly wrong. Kathy and Bill lived on one of the larger hills in town, so she could see much of the town from her driveway. What Kathy saw was shocking.

The sky was pitch-black and filled with rolling clouds. She hadn't been able to hear the rumble of thunder from inside, but now, she heard it loud and clear. And she saw the lighting flashes that were accompanying it. They came crashing down all throughout the town. It was absurd for this time of year, the bitter cold of mid-winter.

It looked like a scene from a weather documentary, but worse. A blinding light, followed by a loud crash, rang out down the street. One of the homes nearby had been struck. Kathy saw that there was no fire. It was Ben's home. He was the neighbor who lived three houses down.

The front porch and front door were charred from the strike. The wind blew away the whiff of smoke to reveal a figure. The figure had to be Ben. He lived alone. His wife had died three years earlier, and he hadn't been the same since. He had turned into a bit of a curmudgeon, but Kathy wouldn't have wished death by lightning on anyone.

The figure started to move. Kathy quickly put her car into gear and headed towards Ben's driveway. She pulled into driveway and, as she undid her seatbelt, she could see Ben standing next to the passenger-side window. She rolled it down. Ben glared at her. He didn't look like himself. He was hunched over, and his face was crumpled into a mean scowl. His skin was ashen, almost blue. His arms hung, apelike, at his side. He snarled at her.

"Are you okay, Ben?" Kathy asked.

"Why don't you mind your own business, Kathy?" Ben said, his face looking even angrier. It was then that Kathy noticed his eyes. They were bloodshot and looked like they were an unnaturally bright shade of yellow.

Ben continued. "You're always sticking your nose in other people's affairs, aren't you, Kathy?" Ben set his hand on the empty passenger-side window frame. He gripped it possessively.

Kathy was scared. This was not like Ben. He was often cranky, but never this outright mean. Kathy silently put her car into reverse.

"Where are you going, sweetie?" Ben asked.

At that moment, Ben's neighbor, Stewart, opened his front door. Stewart was in the midst of a messy divorce. Rumor had it his wife had moved out because she didn't want to deal with his passive-aggressive behavior anymore.

Stewart looked over at Kathy and Ben. "Everything okay over there?" He shouted to be heard above the din of the thunder.

Ben turned around and started walking towards Stewart. He moved like a predator, smooth and strong.

"Do you know why she left you, Stewart?" Ben asked. "Because you're intolerable. You're a pathetic excuse for a salesman, and your love can be easily replaced. She never loved you, anyway."

Kathy was shocked at the boldness of Ben's words. They were mean, rude, and downright hurtful. It was like he was trying to do as much damage with his words as he possibly could. Kathy looked on as Stewart's features went from momentary anger to resigned defeat.

Within moments, another blinding light filled Kathy's vision. *BOOM!* The crash of thunder was instantaneous. Kathy could feel the heat from the strike one house over. The spot where Stewart had stood was blackened and smoking. The smoke cleared, and Stewart was still standing there. He had taken on the same grayish-blue tone and scowling face as Ben.

Ben, halfway across his front lawn, turned and looked at Kathy. His yellow eyes and evil grin told her all she needed to know, and it scared her into action. Kathy pushed the gas pedal and went roaring into the street. Shifting quickly, she sped off.

The next few minutes were a blur. She got out of the neighborhood in two quick turns. All around her were people who looked like Ben. She could see the lightning striking near their homes and cars.

Feeling the pressure all around her, Kathy's pace became more frantic. Every street she turned onto, there were more people glaring and shouting at her. The streets were becoming increasingly difficult to navigate. As Kathy made the final turn onto main street, she couldn't believe what she saw. Cars were strewn all over the road. It looked like the aftermath of an epic blizzard, but there wasn't even an inch of snow on the ground. Each of the abandoned cars was charred from a lightning strike.

There were people standing all over the street. Probably the drivers, which meant they were similar to Kathy's neighbor, cold and mean. Kathy wanted nothing more to do with them.

GROW YOUR MIND SHRINK YOUR WAIST

They were starting to take notice of Kathy. Accelerating through the growing crowd, Kathy realized she needed to get off the road. The architecture of the old library caught her eye, and she made her way towards it. There were only a few windows on the first floor so that seemed like the best place to lay low for awhile. The thumping of hands on the car sent Kathy's pulse through the roof.

Seeing a gap in the crowd, Kathy hit the gas pedal and made it through without running anyone over.

They may be acting weird, but these are still people.

She darted into the library parking lot and hit the brakes. The car skidded to stop, and quick as a flash, Kathy was out of the car and into the building.

As the library door closed, Kathy noticed how heavily she was breathing. She felt dizzy. She stumbled forward and leaned on the front desk.

Yikes, I've let myself go. I ran twenty feet, and I'm out of breath.

As she got her breath back, Kathy noticed movement. She looked toward the entrance and saw something shuffling by the edge of the parking lot. It was moving at a similar pace as the other people Kathy had seen that morning.

PART I: ACTION

Thinking quickly, Kathy opened the half-door separating the counter from the entryway. As she came behind the counter, she nearly tripped on a stack of boxes labeled "Running for Readers 5K." This was the library's annual race to raise money for children in the community. It funded the afterschool reading program that the library hosted.

Kathy started scouring the shelves for a key to lock the entrance door. On the shelf directly underneath the computer, she found her prize. A key with a magnet was stuck to the side of the shelf. Moving silently, Kathy crept towards the entrance. Sticking close to the wall, Kathy was able to lock the door without being seen. She hoped.

Kathy went back behind the front desk and slumped onto the floor.

What now? Where's Bill?

She quickly called Bill and heard his familiar voicemail message.

She dialed her children.

Jacob answered. Things seemed normal by them, but they were keeping their eyes open now.

"Jacob, I need you and Hannah to stay safe and out of danger. Go to the police or the sheriff. Don't stay in those dorms!" Panic came over Kathy unbidden. Her hands felt clammy as she gripped the phone.

"Mom," Jacob said, skepticism sneaking through even though he tried to disguise it. "We're just fine here, Mom. If things are really that crazy out by you, then we'll stay put. Hannah is right here; we're in the dining hall now."

"Jacob, you need to take this seriously…"

But Jacob cut her off. "Mom, I do, but everything here is under control. If things start getting wacky, we'll be ready. We'll be just fine. How's Dad?"

A lump rose in Kathy's throat.

"I haven't seen him since last night. He was up early and out before I woke up. I couldn't reach him on the phone."

"Get that figured out first, Mom. We're going to be all right here. I know you're worried about us, but we're adults now. We'll be safe. We love you, Mom. Go find Dad," Jacob said.

"I love you, too, honey. Tell Hannah I love her, as well," Kathy said.

"I will," Jacob said and hung up the phone.

PART I: ACTION

The silence in the room mirrored Kathy's emptiness inside. She felt fully alone. Each breath that Kathy took sent a quake through her whole body. Her nerves were keyed up so high that small tremors threatened to become big ones. Kathy was on the verge of breaking down.

Her children didn't need her. Kathy grappled with this new reality. She had known for a long time that a moment like this was coming. For their entire lives, they'd needed her. From complete dependence at birth, they had slowly started to grow into more independent and thoughtful people. She could still remember their two-year-old tantrums and attempts at running away as pre-teens.

And now, they were grown. And gone. And she was here, in the middle of a crisis, and she had no one, not even her husband, to lean on.

Kathy took a deep breath.

She tried calling 9-1-1. The line was busy, and the recording on the other end repeated endlessly: *"We are experiencing higher than normal call volume; please remain on the line. If you are in a dangerous situation, please get to safety, and we will be with you shortly. We are experiencing higher than normal…"*

GROW YOUR MIND SHRINK YOUR WAIST

After two minutes of listening to the repetition, Kathy hung up. The chaos of the morning started reeling through her head. The blank, haunting faces of the people she had passed made her hands clammy, and a chill ran up her spine. Kathy's tremors became shakes as her sobs silently wracked her belly. Her husband was gone, her children didn't need her, and the world was going through an apocalypse.

CHAPTER 3
Safe, for Now

*M*inutes had passed by. Perhaps an hour; Kathy couldn't be sure. As she lay on the floor behind the desk, a shadow passed over her. Startled, Kathy let out a shout.

"Oh my!" a shaky voice replied.

"Who are you?" Kathy asked.

"I think the more prudent question is who are *you*? But I'll answer you first. My name is Penny. I'm the librarian."

Kathy looked up. Penny raised an eyebrow, imploring her to answer the same question.

"I'm Kathy. I live on Wood Street. I was leaving for work this morning and…" Her voice trailed off.

Penny let out an audible sigh.

"It's okay," Penny said. "It looks like you're stuck with me here. We've been watching the lightning from the second floor. Things are getting pretty wild out there. Who knows how long we'll have to stay here? The furnace has been having fits lately – just my luck. I have no idea what to do. I'm two years from retirement, and I don't have time for that nonsense out there!"

Penny waved a hand towards the locked entrance and scoffed as she finished her tirade. Then, she turned on a heel to walk further into the library, forcing Kathy to follow her.

They walked up the stairs onto the second level and emerged among a forest of shelving units covered in books. They reached the middle of the stacks, and Penny took a quick right turn. Ahead was an open area; presumably, a leisurely reading space. Around the lounge were three office doors with name placards outside each. Kathy noticed Penny's name on one: **Penny Johnson – Head Librarian**.

One of the doors opened, and two women walked out cautiously. After Penny reassured them that everything was okay, they introduced themselves as Cynthia and Susan.

"What are we supposed to do now?" Cynthia asked Penny.

Susan answered instead. "I'll tell ya what we do: We are going to sit tight until the military gets here and gets things sorted out. We lay low and mind our own business. This is no time for heroics!"

PART I: ACTION

With that, she sat down with a *thud*. Her large, pillowy frame matched the plush, beige couch.

Thankfully, I haven't let myself get that bad…

As soon as the thought crossed her mind, Kathy felt guilty.

I'm sure she's a nice person.

"This would have been a nice time to have a TV in the library," Cynthia said. Her cool, blue eyes darted to meet Penny's. Kathy could sense the bitterness in Cynthia's voice.

Penny's reply didn't do anything to help the mood. "We'd have a TV if people switched it off once in awhile!" Her frustration clearly hinted that this was on old battleground, resurfacing for perhaps the hundredth time.

"Y'know," Susan cut in, "We might not ever get rescued. This could have all hit the White House and spread to the Pentagon, too! Serves them right for running the country the way they have."

"I'll bet the President is holed up somewhere safe. He's probably sipping coffee right now and hanging out in a hot tub. He may have even set this storm loose himself!" Cynthia said with a self-satisfied smile, like she had found a hidden gem of truth.

The conspiracy theories continued on for several more excruciating minutes. Kathy couldn't believe this was what they were talking about. It felt so… unproductive.

So, what if it was a terrorist attack? What could they do about it?

"What if…" Kathy interjected. "What if we tried to lock down the building to make sure nothing from out there can get in? Y'know, board up the windows, block the doors."

Kathy was met with dumbfounded stares.

"We can't do that!" Penny said. "First of all, this building is owned by the city. That would be destruction of public property. Secondly, that is a job that Ben, the maintenance man, would handle. He hasn't checked in yet."

"We should just stay put and wait for someone else to fix this," Susan said.

"Do you really think a bunch of boards will protect us?" Cynthia asked, her voice dripping with sarcasm.

Wow, do these ladies have anything positive to say?

Feeling thoroughly defeated, Kathy resigned herself to inaction. As the day wore on, she became more and more convinced that they were right. What difference did it make what she did?

PART I: ACTION

Kathy was reminded of her time in school. She had always thought of herself as smart. Even when she was young, she'd clung to the idea of being innately intelligent. For her, it had been a way to try and shed the "fat kid" label.

She remembered being afraid to raise her hand in class because the stigma of being wrong outweighed the benefits of having the right answer. If she answered a question and was wrong, everyone would think she was stupid. Even though she was smart, the "fat kid" label was what everyone else saw. And it was what stuck. Kathy knew that it didn't have to be that way. She had seen plenty of her classmates and friends change their lifestyles and become thinner, healthier people. But every time Kathy tried, it ended in failure.

I'm just big boned; there's no way around it.

"No, no, no!" Cynthia exclaimed with a stern look on her face.

Kathy realized she had been daydreaming. The conversation had taken a turn. Cynthia and Susan were discussing the community weight-loss program the library was participating in that year. Each of them was convinced that they had the superior strategy. Kathy had participated in years past with no obvious success.

Many local organizations pushed their members and employees to join the community weight-loss challenge. It was an effort to get people excited about getting into healthier behaviors. Participants weighed in at the start and end of the challenge. The winners were rewarded with cash and other prizes. For the library ladies, each of them already imagining their winnings, a lot was at stake. What had started as a positive conversation about healthy choices had quickly devolved into arguing about the latest diet fads.

As Kathy listened in, she got a firmer sense of their personalities. It was like she was watching a sitcom with each woman filling a different role. Penny was obviously the leader, but she tried not to overexert her authority.

Cynthia continued, "The best way to lose weight is by fasting. Only by getting your body into a fasted state will you be able to burn fat consistently."

Susan scoffed. "So, what you're saying is that for 12 hours or more at a time, I'm not allowed to eat? And once a week, I go a whole day without eating?" Her eyes looked like they might burst from her head. "There's no way I'm doing that!" Susan proclaimed. "I'll take my sausage and bacon in the morning, thank you very much. If you're not getting into ketosis, there's no way you can burn fat effectively. The real secret is limiting carbs, which forces your body to burn fat instead of sugar to function.

PART I: ACTION

You can become a fat-burning machine." Susan crossed her arms smugly as she made her final point.

"Sounds like it's something *you* can definitely use," Cynthia said.

Zing.

Susan's face turned into a scowl.

"You're *both* wrong," Penny chimed in. "I'm doing a 14-day, liquid-only cleanse."

"Gack." Susan made a gagging sound.

"I lost over ten pounds the last time I did it!" Penny replied.

Kathy seemed to remember a time not so long ago when fat was the enemy. She had heard that high-protein diets were the only way to go. But she had also heard that getting too much fat from animal products could lead to cancer. It was all so confusing. None of their plans sounded all that appealing – that was, until they started talking about the amount of weight they could lose.

Maybe I'll give one of them a try...

Usually, when Kathy tried a new diet, Bill was more than happy to participate with her. And he usually lost twice as much weight as she did. It was very frustrating.

Kathy started thinking about Bill.

What had happened to him?

Her imagination ran wild with all the worst-case scenarios. She wanted to curl up into a ball and just go to sleep.

The time came soon enough for that. As it got dark, she and the library ladies gathered near one of the upstairs windows. Looking down at the street, they could see the odd, human-shaped figures prowling about. Once in awhile, she could overhear one of them shouting to the others.

Why won't they leave and go home?

Kathy had told the other ladies about her experience in her neighborhood. With nighttime setting in, none of them were pushing to leave the library.

Cynthia went about finding some sheets in an old utility closet for them to use. Using the couch cushions, they were able to create makeshift beds. The library ladies each set up in their own offices, leaving Kathy in the lounge.

Kathy arranged the furniture into a makeshift fort. It seemed childish, as it probably wouldn't be that effective in repelling invaders, but it calmed Kathy down, nonetheless. She would have to wait until tomorrow to set about finding Bill. She had sent him multiple messages and had gotten no response.

Kathy settled in, not knowing that a bad day was about to get a whole lot worse.

CHAPTER 4
Answers from Above

*K*athy's mind slowly started to ease. The frantic and exhausting pace of the day had taken its toll on her. Kathy's eyes felt dry and tired. Her limbs had taken on a heavy feeling. Kathy glanced at the makeshift fort around her. The pillows and sheets were a purposeful and tangled mess, but it was cozy.

As Kathy rolled into a more comfortable position, she felt the letter Bill had left for her in her front pocket.

I can't believe I forgot about this.

She opened it. It read:

> *"Kathy,*
>
> *I've been short with you. I think it's just work and how tired I am when I get home.*

> *I saw that you left out the flier for that local gym. How about we talk about it over dinner tonight? I'll bring the silverware.*
>
> *Your loving husband,*
>
> *Bill"*

The letter was touching. It tugged on Kathy's heart.

Tonight was supposed to be so different.

Bill was a man of few words. To get him to say anything remotely sweet was like pulling teeth. For him to leave a note was out of character. Kathy couldn't even remember the last time he'd done that.

He had referenced their first date. The waiter had forgotten to bring a spoon for her soup, and he'd disappeared into the kitchen. After waiting awhile, Bill had sheepishly produced a spoon from inside his jacket. He happened to have it on him from his lunch that day. It was such a funny moment that it became an instant connection and inside joke.

I love that man, Kathy thought as the sheet fell to her side and she drifted off to sleep.

PART I: ACTION

Kathy woke up again to shift positions in her uncomfortable makeshift bed. She looked at the clock. 12:40 AM. After a taking a deep breath, she closed her eyes. She heard voices breaking the silence of the night. Soft, but urgent. They steadily got louder. The intensity of the whispers sounded like staccato bursts. Kathy could see a dim light in one of the office windows, the one closest to the public computer section of the library.

It was Penny's office.

Kathy crawled towards the office door, trying to catch what they were saying.

CRASH. CRASH. CRASH.

In rapid succession, the flashes of lighting and crashes of thunder rolled over Kathy. In the briefest of moments, as the lightning flashed, Kathy could see three silhouetted figures.

Oh, no. Is this really happening again?

The dim light from the office was gone.

Kathy stood up a few feet from the closed door. She turned on her cell phone. 37% battery. She turned on the flashlight and brought it up to the office window. Vacant eyes stared back at her as Penny's scowling face came into view. Kathy looked closer. Penny was a troll.

Startled, Kathy dropped the phone and let out a yelp. She quickly grabbed a nearby chair and jostled it between the door handle and the floor, effectively wedging it closed. Upon hearing the noise, Penny – or whatever that thing was – started jostling the door. As quickly as she could, Kathy turned and ran from the office area.

As Kathy hurried through the musty stacks, she could feel her heart beating so loudly that her ears thrummed and thumped with the deep bass of tribal drums on the warpath. Trying to get back to the stairwell, she took one turn and then another.

She was disoriented now. Fear pushed her onward. She caught a glimpse of a glowing exit sign. Kathy made a quick turn and ran smack into the bookshelf.

A shock of pain ran through Kathy's face and knee, the first two places that had connected with the hard metal of the shelving unit. She could feel her body falling in slow motion. She barely felt the impact of the floor. Her vision was cloudy. She couldn't tell if it was from tears welling up or if she had gotten a concussion.

Kathy turned her head to look at the offending bookshelf. A book had been jostled loose after she ran full-tilt into the shelf, and she looked up just in time to see it falling towards her head.

PART I: ACTION

Kathy noticed she was awake.

How long was I out?

Kathy started to lift her head and felt a throbbing headache coming on. She gave up on trying to lift her head for the moment. She brought her balled-up fists to her eyes and tried to rub some clarity back into them.

When she removed her hands, she saw the book. It was a hardcover and had fallen in such a way that it lay open, like she had just taken a quick snooze while reading it.

The hardcover explained her temporary unconsciousness.

Kathy felt around on her head for any bumps or blood. She found a large welt on her forehead. Kathy couldn't tell if it was from the book or from running into the shelf. Either way, it was large. Kathy felt relieved that it was just a bump.

Kathy's gaze fell back to the book. Anger burned inside her. She grabbed the book and prepared to throw it across the room.

"Wait!" a quiet yet firm voice cried into the emptiness of the library. Kathy slowly moved her head and saw nothing.

She began wondering if she'd actually heard anything. She cocked her arm to throw the book again.

"Don't you want to at least know the title of the book that attacked you?" This time, the voice came in crystal clear. It was a woman's voice. She sounded confident and strong. Again, Kathy scanned the room and saw nothing. As her head turned fully to the right, she caught a glimpse of something on her shoulder.

Perched there was a face she recognized. It was the trainer from the exercise flyer she had seen at home. She had clear wings that almost looked like a larger version of a dragonfly's.

No way. Now, I'm hallucinating. I've heard of it happening, but this is something else.

"You're not hallucinating," the small figure replied, as if reading Kathy's mind. Up close, she dominated Kathy's field of view, but she couldn't have been more than six inches high. "My name is Angela. I'm here to watch out for you. There's a lot about the world that you don't know. Right now, what you need to know is in this book."

Kathy heard the distant sound of a door handle jiggling. A bolt of fear ran through her as she remembered the transformations of Cynthia, Penny, and Susan. Kathy quickly propped herself up on one arm and began to stand. A head rush like she had never experienced before came over her. Kathy nearly fainted. She quickly got on one knee and then sat down, leaning against the bookshelf.

"Don't worry about them, Kathy," Angela said, waving towards the office full of trolls. "I made sure that chair wasn't going anywhere!" She winked as she smiled from ear to ear.

Kathy stared blankly ahead until her vision cleared. She glanced at the Angela-fairy. Then, at the book.

First the storm, then the trolls, and now, it looks like I have a fairy godmother. They are going to lock me up in a psych ward if I ever wake up from this.

"You're not dreaming, Kathy," Angela said.

Kathy looked down at the book again.

She picked it up.

Kathy closed the book and looked at the cover. The book was titled, *Necessary Action Required.*

I'll take action, all right. You're getting thrown in a furnace.

She looked at the title again. *Action Required* was underlined in bold red. She opened the book to the first chapter, just to see what it was about. The author outlined how the book would play out, and how a person should look at any situation.

The first point was to DO SOMETHING! The point seemed obvious, but the author elaborated. The reader needed to not just *want* to do something, to not just *talk* about doing something; the reader needed to actually *do* it. As Kathy read on, the author encouraged her to be instinctual, to feel what was most important, and then take action toward that end.

She thought back on the previous day and noticed a pattern. Kathy had taken action quite often in challenging circumstances. On her street, as she was driving, and when she was making those phone calls, she had been decisive and moved towards an end goal.

Things started to change when she had gotten to the library. The women only talked. They talked and talked and talked. By the end of the day, nothing was done. Kathy instinctually knew they needed to secure the perimeter and create a safe haven. Her instincts had been shot down. The expectations of those around her had changed her behavior.

"You've got the idea! Try turning to page 34," Angela smiled as she spoke, clearly excited about the process.

PART I: ACTION

Kathy turned to page 34. The author outlined, *The 3 Keys to Growth: Take action; always learn; know why.* She began to read:

"The core idea of this book is action. Without action, nothing happens. Without it, you remain the way you are, unchanged, as the world around you grows and flourishes. Your stagnation will lead to frustration and unhappiness. You will feel unfulfilled and seek out more trivial pleasures and pursuits. These will leave you feeling temporarily occupied but never fulfilled.

"You were made to crave progress, to thrive on growth. Tony Robbins said it perfectly in a CNBC interview: *There are levels of making it in life, and whatever you think 'making it' is, when you get there, you'll see there's another level. That never ends, because if you stop growing, you're going to be unhappy.'* If you stop growing, you're going to be unhappy.

"Action is the first necessary ingredient to growth; it precedes everything else. Once you've started taking action, you'll begin to see things. You'll see opportunities, and you'll see pitfalls. You'll see doors open that you didn't previously realize were there. As you take action, some of the opportunities will be for learning.

"Learning is the second key to growth. If all you ever did was take action, obstacles would be exhausting. You'd beat yourself against them until you were spent. Learning is often the key to the locked door. As challenges appear in your life, they are like locked doors. You need the right key to get through. Sometimes, action is the key, and you'll be able to pass through. Many times, you'll need to learn something. Especially in moments of failure; learning is your way out.

"Failure can be your greatest teacher. Or it can be your greatest enemy. If you learn from failure, it can take you wherever you want to go. If you are defeated by failure, you'll stay right where you are, tired, jaded, and hiding from life's great adventure. As you learn more about yourself, you'll dig into a deeper meaning and purpose.

"Knowing why is your third and most elusive key to success. Most people never get this key. They'll hit the locked door, struggle to push through it, learn all they can about it, but are left with no progress. Tapping into your deeper purpose and knowing why you're pursuing something will often blow the door wide open. Purpose leads to passion. Passion will motivate you when your reasons run out. It will inspire you when new ideas run dry. It will energize you when exhaustion strikes.

"Your 'WHY' is your superpower. take time to develop it and cultivate it. You'll feel it radiate through you. 'WHY' connects with emotion. Emotions are neither good nor bad. They all have a reason for existing. Like tools in a tool kit, that emotional connection will serve to guide you.

"Your 'WHY' will give you purpose, and that translates to more action and more learning. When all else around you is failing, take the time to ask: WHY?"

Kathy set the book down. She had never thought of her life in those terms before. It didn't seem possible that those three keys could have so much power over her own life.

She thought about the situation she was in. *Why is all this happening?*

After a few moments, she realized she didn't have enough information to answer that question.

She looked to her shoulder. Angela was gone.

Now, Kathy felt the crushing loneliness and isolation of her situation bearing down on her. The companions whom she had known – miserable though they were – had just turned. Her husband was nowhere to be found. And now, Angela had disappeared.

Kathy felt a welling of emotion inside her. Bill. He was all Kathy could think about. She needed to find Bill and make sure he was all right.

Action Lessons

Kathy took a big step in this opening act. She prepared herself to take some major action to change her health. She had the flier, she was ready to make the call, and then, chaos struck, and she was forced to make tough decisions that kept her mind off the future and firmly rooted in the present. Sound familiar?

Most people underestimate the necessity of action. We know deep in our hearts that some things need to change, but we sit on the sidelines and wait for a solution to fall from the sky. Not all of us are as fortunate as Kathy. The answer may not fall directly onto your head. You may need to put in some work. I'll detail four steps to go through as you take action in your life. Most of these happen organically, but if you notice an area you struggle in, it may take extra focus on that step until you can make it into a normal pattern.

There are four major themes within the process of taking action:

- **MINDSET:** *Mindset* influences everything you see and do in the world. If you can shift the way you think, many more possibilities will be open to you. There are two mindsets we'll dive into: The Fixed Mindset and the

Growth Mindset. We'll see how they influence our behavior and perspective, and how to shift from one way of thinking to another.

- **CHANGE:** *Change* is essential if you want to get to a different place in your life. If you don't like your present circumstances, then change will be necessary. We'll explore which changes to make and how to go about it.

- **MOMENTUM:** *Momentum* is built on small actions. When small actions are repeated, they begin to build in power. If you want to feel like you're full-speed ahead on the weight-loss train, it is essential to get that locomotive moving. Not with one Herculean push, but with the consistent application of shovelful after shovelful of coal. If you find yourself "lacking motivation", what you're really missing is the power of momentum. We'll learn how to build it and how to get it to work in your favor, instead of against you.

- **SETBACKS:** *Setbacks* come as part of the package. Don't be surprised when they seek you out. If you spend your time focusing on the injustices of the moment, you'll quickly lose your momentum and find yourself stuck in a plateau. We're going to find out how to deal with setbacks quickly and how to plan for their inevitability.

Mindset

"If success means they're smart, then failure means they're dumb. That's the fixed mindset."

—Carol Dweck, *Mindset*

You need to get into the habit of owning your decisions – and, especially, the outcomes. If you're flabby and out of shape, the first step to fix that is getting real and owning that it is YOUR responsibility. It can be easy to blame an external situation or circumstance. *I'm out of shape because everyone in my family is; it's genetic. I have a short temper because my boss stresses me out; it's not my fault. There was a traffic jam, so there was no way I could have made it on time.*

By taking ownership, you put your mind into a creative and aware state. You start thinking: *What could I have done better to get a better result?* Instead of blaming your circumstances and moving on, you begin to see more opportunities. Many people avoid this type of thinking because the weight of it – especially at first – can feel overwhelming. When you take blame out of the equation, much of the bad and good in life falls squarely on your shoulders. With practice, you will begin to see which aspects of your life are truly circumstantial, and which you have power over. I know you'll find that, in most things, you have a significant amount of control. This thinking shift is the difference between "the fixed mindset" and "the growth mindset".

If you shift the blame in your life, you will never take action to fix your problems. Step one is owning it. Step two is setting boundaries. This is more difficult, because it involves other people. When Kathy arrived in the library, she was speaking with the librarians. Kathy sensed a negative vibe from them. Being stuck in a room full of negative people can be exhausting and truly disheartening. They were able to effectively influence Kathy's behavior for the worse.

There is a powerful force at play in situations like this one. A type of peer pressure that creep in based on the beliefs of those in the group. In psychology, these are known as "social norms". When it comes to negative people, I call it the "crab mentality". The story goes that if multiple crabs are placed in the bottom of a bucket with no lid, a crab may try to escape. When one crab begins to make significant progress towards escaping the bucket, the other crabs will team up to bring that crab back to the bottom.

PART I: ACTION

This happens so often when it comes to fitness. A person will start making real progress towards a goal, and those around them will – oftentimes subconsciously – try to pull them down. They will downplay the significance of their success or make rude comments about a person looking wrinkly, unhealthy, or sick. These comments can seriously derail the forward progress that many of us have built up.

This behavior stems from a mindset embedded so deep that many people are unaware it even exists, or that it can be changed. People who pull others down do so out of a sense of inferiority. They think: *If you are making a good change, that change reflects poorly on me, and I can't have that.* This feeling of inferiority comes from what Carol Dweck calls "the fixed mindset".

The Fixed Mindset

People who are in a fixed mindset believe that their intelligence, skills, and abilities are set. They believe that you're either naturally gifted at something or you're not. People with this mindset value being seen as smart and being called talented. When a fixed mindset person comes across a difficult problem, they will tend to quit early because if they don't get it right away, they must not be "smart enough" to solve the problem.

This mindset is focused on appearances and protecting the ego. Phrases like "I can't do that," "I'm just not good at _____," and "I was bad this weekend" all reinforce the fixed mindset. Let's analyze each phrase:

1. **I can't do that.** The words "I can't" automatically eliminate all other options. There's probably something else you *could* do, but because you aren't priming yourself to think there is, the other options won't show up, and it becomes self-fulfilling. It is true because you *believe* it to be true.

2. **I'm just not good at losing weight.** Here we see a person falling into a logical fallacy. The way something went in the past does not need to define the present and the future for all time. With this phrasing, there is no room to *become* a person who is good at losing weight.

3. **I was bad this weekend.** We all make poor choices at times, but we needn't assign morality to it. If eating certain types of foods leads to "goodness" or "badness", then that means we're trying to keep score. And when it comes to scoring, we always remember the bad scores more than the good scores. Stop keeping score and take positive action instead.

PART I: ACTION

Having said all that, I think you can see that some of Kathy's new "friends" have a fixed mindset. After reading about it, it's easy to shrug this one off and say it's a problem other people have. You've probably found several ways to distance yourself from this idea because it's uncomfortable to think that you may be "one of those people." I assure you, even crazy, growth-minded people have areas in their life where they think with a fixed mindset. Find those areas in your life and start changing the way you phrase things. If you're reading this book, fitness and nutrition is a great place to start.

If you say, "I just can't eat healthy," that is speaking from a fixed mindset.

However, if you say, "I really struggle to eat healthy on weekends," that is speaking from a growth mindset.

The Growth Mindset

Your mindset will change the way you think. It will change the way you behave. The easiest way to get a glimpse of your mindset is to analyze what happens when you come across an obstacle. Growth-minded people will see the obstacle and try to get better at their craft or work harder to get past the obstacle. They may fail or be defeated, but that is not the end for them. In sports, the legends are the ones who grow and get better *because* of the losses they sustained. Coming up short is an opportunity to get better for next time, because there *will be* a next time.

Fixed-minded people, in contrast, will try to find an easier way. Often, they will seek the easy way out. In weight loss, this is typically in the form of a pill or a crash diet program. Competitors with a fixed mindset will avoid tough challenges. They will seek out easy targets to feel better about themselves. At work, they will take credit for work they haven't done and volunteer for the most visible and easiest jobs. This means they can look smart but won't look like a fraud.

Which one are you?

Whichever way you answered, you're right – *and* you're wrong. The general mindset a person has will influence a lot about them. As I mentioned above, even growth-minded individuals will have areas in life where they think with a fixed mindset. For some, it may be foreign language study, going skydiving, or public speaking. A quick way to identify a fixed mindset is the phrase, "I can't." This implies that you not only are incapable in the present, but you are unwilling to try, and will be unable to do so in the future, as well.

PART I: ACTION

When Kathy's new friends were discussing new diet trends, there was a lot of fixed-mindset thinking involved. When they said, "I can't" or "I wouldn't", they instantly limited themselves.

You may be reading this and thinking that your life is full of negativity and bad influences. Your cup keeps running dry. Maybe you've got some bad habits you need to kick. Maybe your friends are major complainers. Maybe you hate the work you do. Perhaps your needs are always last on the list.

You have the power, *right now*, to do something about it.

If your cup keeps running dry, it's up to *you* to figure out how to fill it. I'm going to keep referencing other experts, resources, and ideas as a way to help fill your cup. Exercise and nutrition will become key habits to engage in, but to get consistency and joy in those areas, you will need to look at them from the proper perspective. Without that perspective, they will become too difficult, time consuming, and expensive for you to pursue. With the wrong mindset, they will be too tough for you.

Kathy is in a tough spot in the book right now. She's surrounded by negativity. She feels powerless to do anything in the face of such a monumental change. Kathy represents a piece of all of us. She needs to get out of that situation. You may need to do the same. Think of yourself as a helpless and dependent pet. It's up to you to feed, water, and nurture yourself. Take the time to do it, because you're worth it.

Change

"If you do not change, you can become extinct."
—Dr. Spencer Johnson, *Who Moved My Cheese?*

Kathy started her fateful day with great intentions. It was supposed to be the day things were going to change for the better. We have been in this situation countless times. Right when we're about to make a change on our own, life comes in and scrambles things up. Change is a necessary part of life. It is relentless. It is powerful. It can work for us if we embrace it. If we run from it, it can destroy what we've worked so hard to build.

If we're not growing, we're regressing.

The process of change is constant. The above quote from *Who Moved My Cheese?* is the most difficult thing to see as a fitness professional. People desire different outcomes, but they are unwilling or unsure how to make real change in their lives. Take a lesson from Kathy. If you are not seeking change wholeheartedly, it will come and find you. It might be a heart attack or cancer. It might be missing out on playing with your grandkids because your body is physically unable to keep up with them. It might be waking up one day, and your children have moved out, and you didn't get the chance to be the parent you wanted to be. These are painful moments that none of us wish for.

Kathy is at a transition point in her life. Her kids have grown up and left, and she's grappling with her new reality of a reduced parental role. She is also experiencing a change in the world around her. She recognizes her need for change, but she only has a small idea of how to go about manifesting it.

Rational vs. Emotional

We have two halves in our brains: The rational half and the emotional half. The rational half is logical and eloquent. It reasons and has lots of intricate control. The other half of the brain is emotional. It is a steam engine. It has power, strength, and depth that can move mountains. Chip and Dan Heath describe how both halves interact in their book, *Switch: How to Make Change When Change is Hard*. They describe the left hemisphere of the brain – the rational, intellectual side – as the rider, and the right hemisphere – the artsy, emotional, and imaginative side – as the elephant.

When it comes to sheer force of will, the elephant will win every time. The elephant screams, "I WANT THAT THING!" When the elephant gets hooked, there is no stopping it. Here's an example my pregnant wife and I experienced while on vacation.

I feel that helping people in need is a good thing to do. We have a giving fund in which we'll set aside money to help people. It is usually someone within our network who needs help.

We were in a large city and passed by many homeless people. Most of them had a sign telling their story. (Story connects with us emotionally. It motivates the elephant.) We walked by one woman with a sign that had only had six words on it. It moved my wife to tears, and we donated much more than we normally would have. In six words, this woman's situation touched us deeply. The sign read: *I'm homeless and pregnant, anything helps.*

We were on our "babymoon," which is when a young couple who are expecting their first child go on a vacation to celebrate their growing family and the end of their "freedom" as a couple. Therefore, the story on the homeless woman's sign made a connection to us. It stirred us emotionally, and it got us to take action to help the woman in need.

If you are seeking change in your life, I encourage you to find ways to get both your elephant and your rider engaged, by finding something you can connect to.

PART I: ACTION

Logic and Systems – The Rider

When most people embark on a journey to better health, they say, "It's time to take control!", and they begin to change lots of the problems that they think are bringing them down. Many people can continue in this way for months, even years for some. But at a certain point, it breaks down. There's a snapback. And then, it's all downhill. Most dieters end up heavier than they were when they started their new diet.

Kathy was in this place when she decided to make a call to a gym. She knew it made logical sense to seek help from an outside professional. It was time. As the story continues to unfold, we'll get better glimpses into what works best for Kathy.

I'll give you a little foreshadowing here: Simple is better; sustainable is best. Target small changes that you feel like you could maintain for a lifetime. Your logical mind will get excited because it's making progress and there's planning and systems to create. More importantly, your emotional mind won't freak out because it thinks the sky is falling.

Connect to Emotion – The Elephant

The fitness industry uses two main types of advertising to connect to its customers. The first method, where the advertising will show sexy, scantily-clad people sweating beautifully as they use some bizarre device to "create" their incredible physique, is so overused, it has started to become cheesy. The second method, using testimonials by showing a "before" and "after" picture, along with a story, is one of the most effective ways to get the audience to buy-in.

Here's why these two methods work so well: They appeal to our emotions, not our logic.

Let's start with the sexy spokesmodel. We know that the guy demonstrating the Ab Crunch 3000 machine probably used other methods to get his rippling muscles and abs. Logically, we know it's not the product that got the model to that point, but emotionally, we see two things: The "ideal" image, and the product that will help us get it. Our emotional brain makes that connection, and many of us will take the chance that it will work for them and call right away. After all, they are throwing in not one, not two, but *three* one-pound wrist weights. Are they helpful or useful? Who cares? They're *free!*

The testimonials hook our emotions, as well. We see someone who was once like us, someone who made a change and has gotten the results we wish we could have. They have shown us a way to do it, and that gives us hope. It is proof that it can be done.

PART I: ACTION

These are a couple of ways that advertisers can motivate us to buy their products. Now, I'll show you how to use these same methods to motivate *yourself*.

- **Step 1: The "Before" Picture.** Every great story of triumph has a beginning. If you want your future to look different from your past, you need an inflection point – a point in time when things turned around for good. Commemorate that moment. Capture it as a picture. You probably hate having your picture taken. Good, because that means you're emotionally ready to see that picture and make a change. Get a good headshot and profile shot. This will be your fuel – not of self-hatred, but of self-betterment.

- **Step 2: Check-In and Accountability.** This picture is meant to serve as a trigger – a daily, weekly, or monthly reminder of where you were when you started. If, at first, it is too painful or overwhelming to see yourself like this, then don't look at it until you feel like you've made some headway. It may take 10 to 20 pounds before you can visually see a difference. Don't worry; keep taking positive steps, and you'll see and feel progress. Social media can be a great accountability for many people. Post that "before" picture and make a public statement about your intentions. If that's not your style, get a personal trainer who isn't afraid to challenge you to be better. Look at your "before" picture as often as it's useful for you.

Take the pictures. Go. Do it. Even if they're blurry mirror selfies. This book will still be here waiting when you return. Remember, if you're not willing to take a small step now, how are you going to take the big steps that are necessary later?

Looking for some inspiration? Here are some of our favorite client stories. We take our clients' pictures when they start with us; that way, they can celebrate their change. **https://www.talltrainer.com/blog?tag=transformation+stor ies**

Momentum

"Fear is the mind-killer."
—Frank Herbert, *Dune*

Momentum is an invisible force that can be felt. You intuitively know when momentum is working against you. It is the feeling of not being able to make progress or being stuck in a rut. However, when momentum starts working in your favor, it feels like all you touch turns to gold, and weight loss and healthy behavior is natural and almost easy.

How can you gain momentum?

Action. Action builds into momentum. Taking a step in the right direction has been proven to add confidence and self-satisfaction to our lives. When we do the opposite – stagnate and worry about an action that needs to be taken – we are full of fear. Fear will wreck your momentum and bring your life to a screeching halt. Kathy experiences both momentum and fear in the first few chapters.

When Kathy left her neighborhood and headed for the library, she had momentum. She was making decision after decision. She left the neighborhood, chose the library as a likely safe spot, and made phone calls to her loved ones. Then, fear started to set in. She was afraid of what to do next. This fear was compounded by the interpersonal situation of the librarians, which we talked about in the mindset portion.

Fear will set momentum humming in the opposite direction. Fear will kill creativity and activate your "lizard brain," which houses the deepest and most ingrained instincts baked into our souls: The "fight-or-flight" instinct. When you're living in fear, your frontal cortex – the part of your brain that is responsible for rational and logical decision-making – goes quiet. The best way to get through fear and get into your "right" mind is to *do something*.

Imagine a child poised to jump into a pool. As adults, we know that they will be perfectly safe. If things are a total disaster, they'll get water up their nose and need a nearby adult to buoy them above the water. To the child, the decision to jump begins to grow in importance, and fear begins to set in. The child waits near the edge of the pool, makes a small motion forward, and then moves back from the pool. This can often last for several minutes or more. As adults, we begin to get frustrated. We say, "Just jump in, already!" We recognize the need to take action, to *do* the thing, whatever that thing may be.

I would say the same to you. Just jump in, already! You have enough tools and information *right now* to take a step towards reclaiming your life. You can choose to buy apples at the grocery store instead of cheese crackers. You can cook a larger side of vegetables to go with the meat and potatoes demanded by your family. You can choose to go for a walk instead of watching another TV show.

The secret to building momentum is to keep pushing forward. Those times when it seems like everything is pushing against you are actually the times when you can get the most momentum. When Kathy was pushing to get the library into a more defensible position, she was met with resistance. Were she able to convince the librarians to work on it with her, she would have found a huge boost in momentum. Instead, her momentum came to a screeching halt. Remember, those times when it is toughest to forge ahead are the times that will have the biggest impact.

Take action. Build momentum. Repeat.

Consistency is King

I love this quote by philosopher Will Durant as he summarizes Aristotle: *"We are what we repeatedly do. Excellence, then, is not an act, but a habit."* I'm sure you've heard this quote before, as it has been championed ad nauseum in the personal growth sphere. Yet, it keeps coming up. People keep using it. So, why are we focusing on a trope? Because when you apply it, it works.

We know that momentum can carry us past fear. We know that doing the tough thing in the moment will solidify our resolve. What you may *not* know is that progress is the key to motivation. I see this every day as a personal trainer. We weigh-in daily in our classes – not because we expect daily progress, but because we need data to show progress over time. Monday is usually the toughest day, as many people see an uptick on the scale. Those who made poor decisions and *don't* see an uptick on the scale feel like they got away with something, and maybe they'll be able to sneak by again. Those who did great work and see the scale head in the wrong direction freak out and begin to lose hope.

People expect instant results. They may not consciously think they do, but that thought is just below the surface, waiting to pounce and ruin any momentum they may be building. I tell my clients that the data only matters in a week-to-week comparison, not a day-to-day comparison. If we compare Monday to Wednesday of the same week, there hasn't been enough time for your body to show the changes you've been making. However, if we compare this Monday to last Monday, we'll have a much clearer picture, as many of the small, daily variables that impact your weight have leveled out.

As you work on your journey, you'll need to continue plugging away, every day. The more positive progress days you can string together, the more likely it is you'll get to your big goal. The more consistent you are in your progress, the more motivation you will find. Making a dent in a big project feels good. The more you avoid a project, the scarier it becomes.

If you have a mountain to climb, start by taking one step.

PART I: ACTION

Setbacks

"Just because your mind tells you that something is awful or evil or unplanned or otherwise negative doesn't mean you have to agree. Just because other people say that something is hopeless or crazy or broken to pieces doesn't mean it is. We decide what story to tell ourselves."

—Ryan Holiday, *The Obstacle is the Way*

You are writing the narrative of your own life. That is what Kathy represents in this book: A fictional character with her own story, challenges, and opportunities. She has come so far as a person, and so have you. In many ways, her story wrote itself. It's the oldest story there is: A tale of trial, hardship, and eventually, triumph.

You are in charge of writing *your* story. You get to choose how it goes. When you get to this moment, does the door slam shut? Do you never take the necessary steps to open it? Or does the obstacle become the path forward? Can the most difficult and trying experience you went through transform you into the person you desire to be?

Change and difficulty are where growth lives. Growth makes us happy. If you're unhappy, there's a good chance you aren't growing. Whenever I come to a difficult time in my life, if I can rise up and grow through the challenge, I feel happier and more accomplished. When I run from my challen~~g~~

growth, I feel stagnant, and I undermine myself i~~n~~

also tend to lean on my unhealthy coping mechanisms,

me nowhere.

At the beginning of the story, we see that Kathy is stagnant. She goes through the motions, day after day, not seeing anything happen differently in her life. She's unhappy, but she can't figure out why. The reason, as we've just learned, is a lack of growth. Subconsciously, she knew that something needed to happen. She needed a shake-up. And that's why she latched onto the fitness flyer. It was something that would push her outside of her comfort zone, and hopefully, help her grow.

Before she could even make the phone call to get started on this new journey, her life got turned upside-down. She went through a major setback before she even got started! That's rough! The fact that you are taking the time to read this book tells me a lot about you already. There's a strong chance you have had many setbacks and obstacles keeping you from achieving the results you so desperately crave.

Setbacks tend to follow a pattern: There is the problem itself; there's the pity party that happens after the setback; and then there's the part where you get up, dust yourself off, and keep on keeping on.

PART I: ACTION

The Initial Setback

This is what we point to when we say, "I stopped my diet because _____ happened." Pick your flavor here: A friend passed away; you got swamped at work; one of your kids was in a crisis. There's an infinite number of possibilities. The most important thing to understand here is that on a journey worth taking – whether it is for your health, weight loss, getting stronger, etc. – there *will* be conflict. Have you ever read a good story that didn't have conflict? No, because it would be super boring, and you'd get annoyed.

The same goes for our lives. Conflict and setbacks are inconvenient, to be sure, but they serve the purpose of giving us life and allowing us to focus on something we can overcome. When you overcome an obstacle, you get to be a hero. The bigger the obstacle, the better the story.

For your story, there will inevitably be obstacles. It comes with the territory. Prepare your mind for them. When they pop up, you'll recognize them for what they are: Opportunities.

The Pity Party

After a setback, there is often a "recovery" period. During this period, we have a tantrum, grieve, feel sad, get angry, and experience any number of other feelings. The most important factor here is *time*. You only have a finite amount of time to do things in this life. If you spend most of your time feeling mopey and throwing yourself a pity party every time something doesn't go your way, you'll find that progress will always elude you.

Dave Ramsey, a financial expert who has helped tens of thousands of people get out of debt, said something that I absolutely love: *"Success is a pile of failure. You're just standing on top of it and not underneath it."* If you're seeking success in health and fitness, you need to get out from under the pile. That's what a setback is: A failure.

Failure is difficult to deal with. Often, we bring a lot of emotional baggage with us. When failure happens, we open up the old script, and we begin reciting the sacred words: "I'm no good. I can't do it. It's just not something I'm capable of. I'm a failure."

If you stay in that loop, you'll never get anywhere. I encourage you to fully feel the gravity of your failure. Sometimes, awful things happen to great people. It's important to feel that injustice, to feel sad about something, and to get angry about how unfair it is. Allow yourself to feel these things. And then, focus on the positive and move on.

PART I: ACTION

Back in the Saddle

This concept is so ingrained in us that it has its own set of clichés, depending on your interests. If you ride horses, you "get back in the saddle". If you're a car enthusiast, you "get it back in gear". If you're a farmer, you "dust yourself off".

While clichés are often annoying, they exist for a reason. They have such a strong kernel of truth that they have survived for centuries, sometimes millennia. Where there is a cliché, there is something worth taking note of, because it has stood the test of time.

You've had a setback. You've felt bad about it. Now it's time to get back up and get back to it. The faster you can transition between these steps, the more progress you'll see, the more actions you will take, the more momentum you will build, and the more growth you'll experience. You'll build on these failures, and eventually, you'll be standing on top of them, instead of buried underneath them.

I'm not talking about skipping steps. I'm talking about legitimately working through them. To deny your feelings about a setback means there is fear lurking in you. If you allow fear to live with you, it will continue to trip you up. Oftentimes, people are afraid of facing up to a situation. It can be tough to accept the fact that you had a binge-eating episode. You may be grappling with the idea that you are an emotional eater. Those are hard facts, and they will take some time to digest. But once you come to terms with them, you'll be able to get back up, and you'll stay firmly planted in the saddle the next time an obstacle arises.

The best part about this process is that eventually, obstacles become small enough that you don't lose momentum. They don't knock you flat on your face; they become more of an inconvenience. A hiccup. A bump in the road.

The refractory period after a setback becomes so small that most people don't even see it. You saw the issue, felt the emotions you needed to feel, and moved on. You left it behind and continued on to your glorious future.

PART II

LEARN

CHAPTER 5
Daring Escape

*W*ith newfound purpose, Kathy headed back to the lounge and gathered her things, the shaking door only giving her momentary pause.

In the small window, Kathy could see the trolls' heads, stacked on top of each other like they were in some sort of Three Stooges routine. Their heads kept shifting, and it was obvious that they were pushing each other out of the way to get the best view.

"Let me out, and I'll give you a candy!" Cynthia said.

"I bet you don't have anywhere else to go. Stay here with us!" Susan said, her eyes gleaming under a furrowed brow.

"Nicely done, Kathy; looks like you bumped your head pretty good. With that concussion and your brilliant ideas, the world out there doesn't stand a chance," Penny said sarcastically.

Deceit, sarcasm, and negativity spewed from their scowling faces. Kathy felt icky inside. Grabbing her cell phone off the floor, she quickly left the lounge. Their taunts and jabs nipped at her as she moved towards the stairwell to the bottom floor. The sweat on her body was cold. She felt drained and jumpy. Kathy brushed the nerves aside.

I need to find Bill. No one else is looking for him; it's up to me.

Kathy arrived at the bottom floor near the front desk. The light near the entrance was dim. As Kathy looked outside, she could see a few silhouettes of what must have been people.

Let's call it like it is. Those are trolls.

Kathy took a quick inventory. Jacket,. Gloves. Hat. Boots. Phone. Keys. Book.

That ridiculous book. She was still carrying it. She set it down and turned to walk outside. She remembered her interaction with the fairy.

That book must have been important.

Kathy dashed back to the counter and grabbed it. Book in hand, she strode out into the darkness.

PART II: LEARN

Keeping close to the shade of the library, Kathy looked out over the landscape. It was very dark with only the sliver of a moon providing any light. The light it *did* produce was dim and created dark shadows next to the buildings. Kathy glanced at her phone. It was at 28% battery. She looked at her messages. Bill had not responded to any of the texts or calls she had made.

Not a good sign.

Bill did shift work at an industrial complex uptown. If he was gone before she woke up, it meant he was headed to work early that day. Heading uptown would be her best chance to find him.

Starting her car would be too noisy and would leave her totally exposed. Staying in the shadows, Kathy moved from building to building. As she travelled, Kathy's heartrate began to drop. The trolls in the library had gotten Kathy more stirred up than she had first realized. The cool, crisp air was almost silent. If she hadn't known better, she'd have thought it was a beautiful night.

Things are going to be okay.

Three blocks from the industrial complex, Kathy spotted Bill's car. It was abandoned but showed no signs of damage. That was a good sign. It was still disconcerting. The car was angled away from her, so she could only see the rear of the car and the passenger side.

Kathy crept closer. She rounded a corner and ran smack into a body. Scared out of her wits, Kathy let out a yelp. As the sound left her lips, she tried desperately to stifle it. But it was too late.

The body she ran into turned to face her. The face was bunched up in what looked like a cross between a scowl and a frown. It was definitely a troll. And it was definitely reaching for her!

"Come here, my pretty!" the troll said.

As Kathy's yelp echoed through the street, she turned to run. Turning back around the corner she had come from, Kathy could see trolls headed in her direction from all around. Her only hope was to get to Bill's car.

Kathy ran. She'd never considered herself a runner, but today, she felt like an Olympian. Her muscles pulsed as she launched each leg off the ground. The car came closer and closer. The trolls around her were closing in. Thirty yards. Twenty yards. Ten.

A few yards short of the car, Kathy found herself surrounded on all sides by a horde of trolls.

A hand grabbed her.

And then another. And another.

Kathy squirmed and screamed, knowing that this was probably the end, hating that she was going to turn into a troll just like the rest of them.

The trolls were taunting her now. They said things that cut to the core, the things she whispered inside her own head when she was full of doubt.

"Don't resist, Kathy. You know deep down, you're not strong enough to save yourself."

"You'll never amount to anything."

"You can't do it."

"Who do you think you are?"

"I'm just trying to save my husband!" Kathy yelled.

As they spoke, more of the trolls' hands came in to restrain her.

She expected pain. Other than inner turmoil, Kathy felt nothing. She started moving more, trying to break free. The hands gripped harder, and more appeared from the wall of bodies to hold her down.

She looked up to see a crowd around her. She felt like a football, surrounded by strong figures, held in place. She could sense the power and energy around her, but she was unable to move. She was waiting for a change, something to set her free. It didn't come.

She bucked again, trying to break loose from the iron grips. Any time she threw off a hand, another one came in to replace it. The trolls above her all looked the same in the dim light. Sad. Empty. As they spoke, she could see fiendish delight in their expressions. They enjoyed tormenting her. And harder yet, some of these trolls used to be her friends. They didn't care about her now.

"You'll never save him."

"What's a run-of-the-mill lump like you doing trying to be a hero?"

"You're only delaying the inevitable by fighting. He doesn't really love you; that's why he hasn't come back."

Kathy struggled and raged against their grip for what felt like hours. The lining of her jacket was caked in sweat, and she was exhausted. Unable to fight back anymore, Kathy relaxed. Her muscles ached, and her will to fight was sapped.

She lay on the ground, waiting for whatever was going to happen, resigned to her fate.

What happened next surprised her.

PART II: LEARN

Thunder rumbled in the sky above her. Kathy noticed the sky above her darkening, like a stray storm cloud had come to hover directly over her. The cracks of thunder grew in volume and intensity.

The trolls released their grip and backed up. They were chanting now:

"You'll. Never. Save. Him."

"You'll. Never. Save. Him."

"You'll. Never. Save. Him."

As the trolls backed up into a large circle, Kathy caught a glimpse of her husband's car. She was at a different angle than before. She could see the driver's-side door. It was charred and black. He had turned.

Kathy looked around the crowd, trying to identify a face. The gnarled faces all looked foreign and unfamiliar now.

The storm and the chanting were reaching a crescendo. The cloud above her was descending. Kathy knew what was going to happen next. There would be a bolt of lightning, and she would become one of them. Kathy no longer cared.

As Kathy ran these thoughts through her head, she noticed two trolls moving towards her. They were far outside the circle, but closing in rapidly.

"You'll never save him. You'll never save him. You'll never save him."

Kathy could feel the electricity in the air. She could smell the ozone produced by the cloud. She closed her eyes and waited.

"Outta the way!" a man's voice yelled.

She opened her eyes and saw the two trolls who had been moving towards her. They were shoving their way through the circle. They both reached down, and in one fluid motion, hauled Kathy to her feet.

Kathy caught a glimpse of their faces. Definitely not trolls. The scene was chaos. The thunder rumbled louder. The trolls were all yelling a cacophony of insults:

"You can't save her!"

"You're too late!"

"You're outnumbered!"

The new arrivals lifted Kathy's arms over each of their shoulders and began running at full speed to the opposite end of the crowded circle. They lowered their shoulders and charged through the mass of trolls, then came out on the other side without stopping. They sprinted at full speed for over a minute with the trolls in hot pursuit.

They came to the closest building. A door quickly opened for them. They dashed inside.

The door closed with a *thud*.

CHAPTER 6
A New Friend

The fresh scent of lavender essential oils greeted her as she stepped into the dark, unfamiliar space. She felt the tickle of a sneeze that was just out of reach. The man and woman guided her into another room. The lights flicked on. Temporarily blinded, Kathy blinked and wondered what would happen next.

The woman's voice echoed through the mostly empty room.

"My name is Michelle. You're lucky. You were minutes away from becoming one of them." Michelle paused and looked deep into Kathy's eyes. "You could feel it, couldn't you? That hopeless and empty feeling. Like you've been drained of all energy and the will to continue."

"Yes..." Kathy felt herself whisper under her breath.

The man chimed in now. "You understand what's going on, don't you? Those people out there..." The man pointed vaguely at the door. "They are possessed. It must've been the cell phones.

Those things go after anything that moves or does anything with purpose. They exist to shut out the good things in life. Smiles, happiness, productivity. All of it. They grab hold and just don't let go. It's like they can suck out your soul..."

The man's eyes were downcast as his voice trailed off.

"That's enough, Kevin," Michelle said. "We can't be sure of any of that. All we know is that once they grab hold, they don't let go. They only move on once their victim starts acting like them. They're like big bullies."

"Thank you for saving me," Kathy said softly.

The man, Kevin, snapped out of his reverie. Then, Kathy heard it. Footsteps.

A door across the room opened. Silhouetted in the frame was a woman. She stepped forward, the light of the room illuminating her face and her strong physique. Kathy felt like she recognized the woman, but she was not sure from where.

My fairy godmother?

"I'm Angela. Right now, you're in my gym. It's the safest place I know."

Right then, it clicked. Kathy recognized the woman now. She was normally wearing exercise gear. She had all kinds of ads in the newspapers, on TV, and even on social media. Kathy even remembered part of Angela's marketing slogan.

"It's time to take care of you..." Kathy began.

A smile came across Angela's face. *"...and we're here to help,"* she finished. "You're in the right place, friend. Our space here isn't much, but it's safe from the dangers outside. What's your name?"

"Kathy."

"And what's your story?"

Kathy sat upright. She was unprepared for such a direct question.

"Well," Kathy started, "I woke up late for work yesterday, and when I came outside... everything was different."

"It's different for all of us now," Angela said.

Kevin and Michelle nodded solemnly.

Kathy continued, "I stayed at the library; the ladies there were so negative. It was awful. That night, they changed. I had to get out of there. I had to..." A lump caught in Kathy's throat as she thought of Bill. "...find my husband," she finished.

Her right hand moved from her lap to touch her pocket, where the letter from her husband was stashed. Tears sprang unbidden into her eyes.

Angela looked her in the eyes. "We are going to find your husband. And somehow, some way, we are going to cure this epidemic." The seriousness and sincerity with which she spoke convinced Kathy that these things would come to pass. She knew that despite all odds, they would prevail.

What Kathy did not realize was how much she would need to grow and change before she could be reunited with Bill.

"Let's pack it in for tonight. You're under no obligation to stay here, but I recommend at least staying the night until you get your bearings. We've got some blankets and throw pillows you can use."

Kathy thanked her and settled in for some much-needed sleep.

Kathy woke up, disoriented. She felt like she had barely slept. Searching her surroundings, Kathy noticed the exercise equipment and the other people nearby. It hadn't been a bad dream.

The rest of the group began stirring and sitting up. For a late night, Kathy was shocked at how early everyone was waking up.

PART II: LEARN

Angela walked into the room with breakfast. The meager meal of a power bar and fruit was made better by the company it was shared with. Kathy got the distinct sense that these were all good people. Her nerves started to settle down.

Angela took Kathy on a tour of the immediate area. She saw the main exercise room, the small-but-tidy office, and the odd door that Angela told her connected to the restaurant next to them. Kathy loved the feel of the place. It was vibrant with sharp colors and a woman's touch. She especially loved the phrases on the walls: *"There is no 'I can't'."; "Work Hard. Do Your Best."; "Know WHY. Take ACTION. Always LEARN."*

When Kathy's eyes saw the last quote, her whole body turned to see it. It seemed so familiar.

Angela smiled. She reached into the satchel she was carrying and pulled out the book that Kathy had found in the library. Kathy was in shock. She thought she had lost it when the trolls were holding her down.

Angela gently ran her hand across the cover, feeling the raised letters of each word. *Action Required.* She opened to the index and then quickly flipped to a page.

"This book saved my life," Angela said matter-of-factly. "It changed me in a deep and profound way."

Without waiting for a response, Angela started reading:

> "You started this book by taking ACTION. You were decisive enough to start reading, and maybe you even applied some of the ideas. But you probably came up with more questions than answers. You probably failed. And that's okay. The most important thing you can do is dust off after the failure. Failure is the greatest teacher you will ever have. Failure is a gift. If you aren't failing, you are stagnant, and change is coming for you, whether you are prepared or not. The title of this book is *Action Required* because that is the most important step to take. But if it's all you ever do, you will never achieve your true goal. You need two other ingredients: You must know WHY, beyond all shadows of doubt, and so deeply that when you have a choice of an action to take, it will be an obvious decision. The other step in this repetitive process is to LEARN. This is where that failure benefits you. Without learning, your failures will bring you crashing back to the unstable ground of life. If you aren't clear on why you're doing it, that ground becomes impossible to get up from. The

failures break you. When you know why, you can get back up. When you take action again, it's okay if you fail. You'll learn, lean into your 'WHY', and you'll take action again, better prepared for success and always hungry for the reason you're here: Your purpose."

Kathy stood, motionless, trying to digest the torrent of new ideas and perspectives. It seemed to be contrary to everything she had ever learned. Failure was *bad*. Sure, action was important, but thinking and weighing options was what made humans great.

Angela spoke again. "There's a lot there to digest. It will make more sense if I tell you my story.

"Ten years ago, my life was in crisis, and I couldn't figure out why. I felt that nothing was going particularly wrong, but things were unraveling. My marriage was at an all-time low, my career that I had worked so hard to build seemed to be stalled, and I didn't recognize the stranger who greeted me in the mirror. I felt flabby and unattractive. I didn't have my confidence. When the alarm went off in the morning, I just wanted to crawl under the covers and shut out the world. Things were not good. And then, they got worse.

"On a Monday in late Autumn, I was escorted from my job with minimal explanation and zero empathy. I was shattered. I had put so much of myself into that career. I'd identified with it. It was rejection of the deepest kind. I was such a mix of emotions: Anger, anguish, regret, shame, depression. I started sleeping in until 1 PM. My husband became more distant, as he didn't know how to help me. After three months of that, things were nearing a breaking point."

Angela took a deep breath. Her eyes fixed on Kathy's. "I wish I could tell you the answer just came to me one day. That the right book dropped off the shelf and onto my thick head."

Kathy's eyes went wide, and she turned a bright pink. Instinctively, she tried to avoid eye contact.

Angela picked up on her discomfort. She held up the book. "Where did you get this?" Angela asked.

"When I was at the library... it fell on my head as I was trying to figure out what to do," Kathy said, more than a little bit embarrassed.

Angela's blue eyes went wide as her face lit up with a grin. "You're telling me the book you needed fell from the sky right when you needed it?" She whistled. "God must have big plans for you! And you must be way more stubborn than I am!" Her laugh put Kathy at ease. She was so genuine. Kathy decided she could be trusted.

Angela's smile remained as she continued her story. "I wasn't quite as lucky as you were. I decided that I needed to do something. So, as I struggled to send out a job application each week, I stopped by the library and found a few books from the self-help section.

"I got about fifty pages into the first two, and they weren't helpful. They kept talking about putting things out into the universe and spirit energy. Self-help talk like that didn't resonate with me. The third book was different. It was practical and pointed to the exact areas where I needed it most. *Action Required* started me on a journey of self-discovery. I learned and changed more in that year than I had in any year previous – other than maybe age 13; my goodness, puberty was so awkward," she added with a wry smile.

"I took that book and applied it. Day after day, week after week. My progress was slow, but my perspective began to change, and as that happened, I was empowered to make my reality match it.

"I had no idea how to heal the chasm that had opened up between my husband and me. So, I opted to tackle something I knew I could control: Myself. I started working out. At first, I had no idea what I was doing. I remember showing up at a gym and getting signed up. Once I got past the main desk to the gym floor, I had no idea what to do. I saw some people running on the elliptical. I saw people using all sorts of bizarre machines and picking up heavy weights, doing these complicated-looking exercises. They all looked like they knew exactly what they were doing. As I stood there, people were moving past me, and I felt like I was in the way. I was so overwhelmed that I turned around and left. It's so embarrassing to tell that story now, being who I am, but it helps me understand where a lot of people are at. I really know what it's like to be a total newbie and terrified of change.

"I decided that I needed to learn. I hired a personal trainer and started going through the machines and exercises that I saw all the others doing. She was awesome and really helped give me perspective on what to do to get healthier.

"Fitness was a revelation for me. When I started to change my body, my mind changed as well. As my mind got stronger, my body followed suit. It was like a virtuous cycle. I loved the rush I got at the end of a workout. My trainer made it fun and exciting. Even the hard work had its own kind of immediate reward. I was proving to myself, over and over, that my actual limits were way further than I initially believed.

"As I gained control of my body, I started reclaiming other areas of my life. I took responsibility for my share of the problems in my marriage. I owned it 100%. And that was very hard, especially at first. It felt like so many of the issues were my husband's fault. But we were able to come together and rebuild our relationship even stronger, because I took responsibility for what was in my power.

"I had such a profound life change that I decided to pursue a career in fitness. I knew that the way I changed could help thousands of others to grow and change, as well. That's why I started Downtown Fitness Studio. I knew that this process could change lives, build self-confidence, and help others heal."

Kathy noticed she had been staring. Angela's story had touched something deep inside Kathy: Her burning need for connection; the loss of control when her children left; her isolation in a marriage that had lost its intimacy. All of it came bubbling up from the depths. They were feelings that had been compartmentalized and ignored for too long.

"That is quite the story!" Kathy replied. There was a thickness to her voice that she hoped didn't betray her inner emotions.

"It is," Angela replied. "But, so is yours. What's your story? Why are you trying to find your husband?"

"Because I love him. I'm seeing now that we have a lot of work to do on our marriage. He wrote me a letter the morning he disappeared." Kathy paused to remain in control of her voice. "He said he wanted to work on us. I want to work on us, too."

"I think it's awesome that you want to reconcile. Let me ask you this: Why do you want to repair your relationship?" Angela asked.

At first, Kathy was annoyed. *Who is she to question my motives?*

Kathy thought about it for a moment. The question was a deep one. Her facial expression softened.

"I love him. I need him. I'm broken without him." Kathy shocked herself as the last words left her mouth. *Where did that come from?*

"I know we just met each other, Kathy. I want to phrase this delicately. It sounds like you feel things are not working as they are," Angela said.

Kathy nodded.

"You want to fix them. You feel like, by working on the relationship, it will make you whole."

Kathy nodded, slower this time, sensing that Angela was about to make her point.

PART II: LEARN

"Two broken people do not make a healthy relationship. No matter how hard they try, they are still two broken pieces that need to be fixed before they can come together. You need to fix yourself before you can hope to fix the relationship. Now, tell me your story. Your *real* story."

Kathy gulped. Her heart raced, and her palms were sweaty. Her fingertips felt ice-cold, and goosebumps raced up her spine.

Kathy clenched and unclenched her jaw, deciding what she should share and how vulnerable she should be with this stranger.

CHAPTER 7
Attempting Vulnerability

*K*athy's first instinct was to share just a bit of her story with Angela. She had opened up, after all; it was only right to share with her, too.

"My childhood growing up was wonderful. I have great parents who took wonderful care of me. I love them dearly, and I'm thankful to have them," Kathy started.

"But…" Angela prompted.

"But they weren't perfect. I can remember a few times that really left an impression on me. Some of them seem so small, but they devastated me at the time. I can remember my parents telling me I needed to be more careful about what I ate.

"It always seemed like my mom was on some sort of new diet. So, I started trying it, too. I'd get so hungry, this feeling of need and emptiness welling up inside me. I'd ignore it for as long as I could. Then, I'd binge. I must've been six or seven when this was going on. I remember my mom coming into the locked bathroom, where I was bingeing on candy corn. I can barely remember anything from that age, but this memory is burned into my brain. I just remember feeling so ashamed."

Kathy looked down at the floor and cleared her throat. This was already more than she had intended to share. She had told Angela enough to be more than polite. Something inside her tugged at her, a crushing feeling, the fear of being known. Was it also the fear of betrayal?

What if I share it all, and I'm rejected?

Against the fear in her heart and the voice in her head, Kathy continued, "That shame stayed with me. I went through cycles of dieting, bingeing, and I even tried purging. In high school, I was probably forty pounds overweight. People would say to me, 'You have such a pretty face; it's a shame you're overweight.'"

Angela's eyes bugged out, and her jaw dropped open in disbelief.

"Yes, a girl in my high school actually said that to me," Kathy continued. "This same girl and one of her friends from the cheerleading team took me on as a pet project. They showed me how to dress better and do my hair. Then, they showed me how they stayed thin. After a meal, they would go to the bathroom and put a finger down their throat to get the food to come back up. They called it 'pulling the trigger'. I tried it a few times, but thankfully, I wasn't able to master the technique. They abandoned me soon after that.

"High school was hard for me. I knew my parents loved me, but I never felt like they cared enough to really get to know me. They'd ask me how I was doing; I'd give them surface-level responses. They accepted it and moved on. I always hoped that they would see through that. That they would sit me down and just really listen to me. Hear me out without trying to correct me or lecture me. Just get to know me. But they never really did. They always had too much going on. They were too self-absorbed to get to know me. There were other problems and fires to put out."

"What happened to you wasn't fair, Kathy," Angela said. "I think you're beautiful just as you are."

Kathy's first instinct was to brush off the compliment.

"I truly mean that. You are beautiful," Angela repeated.

Angela let silence hang in the air for a moment to allow the words to sink in.

It had the desired effect. Kathy was grateful that she'd meant it. The other voice in her head – the voice that never had anything positive to add – had already started to poke holes in Angela's words. She couldn't be beautiful; she was average-looking. Even if she lost weight, she'd still have baggy skin. Her eyes were too far apart.

Kathy had a moment of clarity.

"Angela, do you ever feel like you have a battle going on in your mind?"

Angela tilted her head quizzically.

"You know, like a battle between good and evil, truth and lies. I feel like I have this voice in my head. It's always so loud and convincing. It tries to tear me down. It says the most awful things, makes me feel terrible. It started running amok after your compliment. In the silence of that moment, I could hear it running wild. And I realized something: It's not *me*."

Angela nodded. A tender smile appeared on her lips.

"It's other people. It's the voices of the people who have put me down. The ones who have left the deepest scars: My parents, former friends, even my husband."

"There's another voice in there," Angela said. She reached out and touched Kathy in the center of the chest with her index finger. "There's a smaller voice that comes from here." Angela's hand returned to her own chest, and she patted it three times. "Call it your inner child. Your true self. Your spirit. God. That voice speaks the truth. But it is so quiet. *So* quiet. It takes a lot to listen to that voice. The other voice is shouting lies so loudly, it often overpowers it. As often as you can, be quiet and listen to that voice. It will steer you right."

Kathy could see tears in Angela's eyes. "Thank you for sharing," Angela said. She reached out her arms and held Kathy's hand.

Kathy started tearing up, as well. "Thank you for listening."

"You've overcome a lot just to be here today. I'm so proud of who you are. And I know that there is a deeper level to you. I know you are capable of more than you've been doing. I want to help you, Kathy. We can't control the world out there," Angela said. "But we can control ourselves. So, let's focus on that and do it to the best of our ability. Then, we can see about saving your husband and getting out of this mess."

Angela looked Kathy dead in the eyes. "You're at a crossroads, Kathy. You can keep doing the things way you've always done them, or you can make a change. One option means hiding and barely clinging to life; the other means growing, finding your husband, and seeing what we can do about this mess out there.

CHAPTER 8
Getting Stronger

*K*athy was starting to wonder whether she had made the right choice. The sweat beaded and dripped from her forehead. Her body ached in places she didn't know existed. All she wanted was a pizza and a day off. And for this plank to end.

Oh, please, Lord, let this plank end. I'll never eat pizza again if this could just be over.

The timer sounded, and immediately, Kathy sank into a pile on the floor.

Ugh, I guess that means I have to follow through.

The variety and difficulty of the exercises varied from day to day. Angela was insistent that they exercise daily, even if it was lighter exercise with more of a focus on stretching. They lifted weights, pushed sleds, rode stationary bikes, and rowed. Goodness, they rowed *a lot*.

It had been almost a week since Kathy had joined the group, and she was ready to give up on the whole exercise thing. It seemed like all it did was cause her pain.

She watched Kevin and Michelle interacting with each other during each workout. It was clear that the couple shared a special bond. She wondered what made them different.

Today's workout was wrapping up. Kathy breathed a sigh of relief and couldn't help but smile. Today had been a tough one.

"Hey, you made it through your first week!" Kevin exclaimed.

Kathy's smile turned into an ear-to-ear grin. Angela and Michelle came over to exchange high-fives with her. Kathy felt so good that she barely noticed the stinging feeling left behind in her palms. The slow, burning feeling in her abs told her that she would be feeling that workout for a bit.

"Great work this week, Kathy. I'm so proud of the changes you're making. I can't wait to see what else you're capable of!" Angela said. "Lets get cleaned up and meet back here for breakfast in thirty minutes. We'll go over today's game plan after that."

So far, this week, the group had raided the restaurant next door for food and taken stock of what they had available. They had painted a large tarp that said, *"THERE IS HOPE"* and put it on the side of the building. Watching from the safety of the roof, Kathy had seen the trolls try to tear it down. Thankfully, it was several feet out of reach – even for the tallest among them. Clearly, they didn't appreciate the encouraging words.

The plan for today was to go out and safely explore the area. The goal was to find food and other people who were like them. Kathy slipped on her coat. As each arm went into its respective sleeve, Kathy could feel her muscles stretch and ache from the week's work. It was annoying, but it felt like progress. As she put her boots on, Kathy's legs quaked. That wasn't from the workout; she was nervous. She had a momentary flashback to her last encounter with the trolls, out in the cold, when she was ready to give up.

Kathy took a deep breath and followed the others. The snow crunched underfoot. The eskimos had over one hundred different words to describe snow. Kathy felt like her home state, New York, was on its way there, too.

Their group was small, only four strong. There had to be more survivors. More people who had fought to keep their positivity.

Angela selected a neighborhood that lead back into town. The plan was to search each house as quickly and quietly as possible.

If things went south, the plan was to meet up at the restaurant next to the gym.

Angela and Michelle were out front. Kevin followed. They were careful to walk with an aimless stagger, slowly weaving their way toward the first target.

The first house looked vacant. As they converged on the side of the house, Kathy looked into the kitchen. The cabinetry was oak, and the marble countertops gleamed in the mid-morning sunlight. The house looked spotless.

I don't know if that's a good sign or a bad one.

Michelle tried the back door. It was locked. The town they lived in was small, and crime was low. Kathy knew many people didn't bother to lock their doors. Kathy was getting a good feeling about this house.

Angela flipped over the welcome mat and found a spare key. She inserted it gingerly into the door handle and turned the key. Silently, the door fell open as the cold air hungrily tried to occupy the warm mudroom.

They entered single-file. Kevin closed the door behind them. *THUD.*

Kevin's eyes went wide as he mouthed the words, *I'm sorry.*

They waited for a few tense minutes. After they were sure there was no sign of life in the house, Angela opened the door that separated the mudroom from the kitchen.

They crouched and tiptoed through the kitchen. They went through an open doorway into the living room.

"Stop right there!" a man's voice shouted.

The lights flicked on, and two people emerged from a small office.

"We've got weapons, and we're not afraid to use them!" a woman's voice intoned.

Both of them clearly looked like they were ready for business. The man had a white handlebar mustache and wielded a titanium baseball bat. The woman wore a scowl underneath fiery-red hair and an intimidating-looking 9-iron.

"We don't mean any harm." Angela spoke for the group. "My name is Angela. These are my friends. We're looking for food and more survivors."

"You're trespassing," the man said.

"We're sorry," Angela continued. "We're from the gym down the road – Downtown Fitness Studio."

"Are you that woman who keeps sending us junk mail? The one that is on TV sometimes?" the woman asked. Her aggressive stance relaxed a bit.

"That's me!" Angela replied with a bright smile. *"It's time to take care of you; we're here to help."*

The woman lowered her club. "John, this is the place I keep telling you I need to go to. She's a nice person; she donates some of her company's profits to charity each month."

John held his bat at shoulder-height for a moment longer. The woman's stern glance motivated him to lower the bat to his side.

"They're still trespassing…" John mumbled.

"Well, they are guests now," the woman said. "My name is Mary, and this is my husband, John. He's been talking all week about what he's going to do if one of those crazies out there tried to get in here."

"We're not crazy," Kathy blurted out.

"I'm not so sure about that," Mary said. "You have to be *some* kind of crazy to workout with *this* lady." She pointed at Angela. "And *another* kind of crazy to come into someone else's home. But you're not like the rest of those things out there, that's for sure."

"We've been calling them trolls," Michelle said. "They are mean, and their scrunched-up faces make them look like some sort of monsters."

"This is Kevin and Michelle; they used to work for me before all this happened. They are the most reliable and trustworthy people I know." Angela gestured to Kevin and Michelle on her right. They both grinned, thoroughly enjoying the compliments.

"This is Kathy," Angela said, her lips curling into a mischievous grin. "She doesn't know it yet, but she's the toughest person to ever walk into my gym."

Kathy blushed. *Does she really think that about me?*

"We want to find more people like you; it's becoming a dangerous world out there. I think it's safer if we band together and pool our resources. Will you join us?"

Mary and John looked at each other. After a brief pause, John gave one nod.

"We're in," Mary said. "As long as I can get a membership to the gym." She broke into a deep belly laugh. The rest of the group smiled.

"Careful what you ask for…" Kevin said.

GROW YOUR MIND SHRINK YOUR WAIST

Every day started the same way. Kathy's first action every day was to check her phone. Maybe today would be the day a message from her husband would be waiting for her. Day after day, the phone was blank. She still communicated with her kids, who were doing just fine. After Kathy checked her messages, she cleaned up her bedding and got ready for the morning.

Everyone filtered into the main gym area by 7 AM. There was Kevin and Michelle, the long-term veterans of the group. Mary and John were settling in well. They weren't the new additions anymore. Tammy was the newest member of the group. She had seen the sign outside and found a side door to bang on and ask for help.

It had been three weeks now since the storm had come into the town and turned the world on its head. The thunder was intense that first day, which only illustrated how many people had changed into trolls. The thunder was much more sporadic now. Kathy only heard it a few times per day. It reminded her of *The Hunger Games*, with each concussive blow signaling that another contestant had perished. These people weren't dying, but was their fate any better?

As Kathy made her way to the rest of the group, she could see Angela packing up her journal. It was one of her many small habits that Kathy had come to notice. Each morning, Angela was up before the sun rose. Kathy only found this out because of a late-night bathroom trip a few days earlier. Since then, Kathy had watched silently as Angela diligently woke up and performed the same ritual, day in and day out. It seemed to involve some form of meditation or prayer, followed by some yoga, and writing in her journal.

Kathy wasn't exactly sure why she was so curious about Angela's morning ritual.

I just don't understand how she has it so together.

That was it. Since Kathy had arrived, Angela had been cool, calm, and collected through all sorts of minor and major crises. The world seemed to be falling apart, and Angela always had a plan. Kathy couldn't imagine how one person could be so put together under such circumstances. It seemed impossible. And yet, there she was.

Is she really a fairy godmother?

"Let's get started," Angela said. The troupe was assembled. Today's workout was high-intensity intervals interspersed with light strength training. It was difficult. Even though the weights were a little lighter than the ones Kathy had used on other days, they felt just as challenging. Kathy had been waking up sore every day. The first week had been the worst. If this wasn't the only safe haven Kathy knew of, she'd have been gone long ago.

Yet, after three weeks, Kathy was beginning to feel better. She was certainly sleeping better at night, and she found it much easier to stay focused during the day.

The workout wound down into some light stretching. As they stretched, Angela walked them through the plan for the day.

"The restaurant doesn't have unlimited food supplies. Eventually, they will run out. We haven't been able to reach anyone with knowledge of what is going on. All the TV channels are dead, and there are no radio broadcasts. We have to assume no help is coming."

Kathy found herself nodding with the rest of the group. That all made logical sense so far.

"We need to secure more supplies, and while doing so, we can scout out our surroundings to see if there are any more people out there who haven't... changed."

They packed lightly and selected a supermarket down the road to investigate.

I hope Angela knows what she's doing.

Learn Lessons

Vulnerability is a Superpower

"Vulnerability is the birthplace of innovation, creativity and change."
—Brené Brown, Author of *Daring Greatly*

Faking It

Faking it will get you nowhere. Yet, we are all so tempted to do it. We try to impress others. We wear masks that we think will make people like us because we're afraid that we're not good enough on our own. To be ourselves and be rejected is too painful. It is much easier to live with the constant sting and abrasion that comes from wearing the wrong mask than it is to risk being seen and rejected.

The fear of rejection is one of the most powerful psychological forces we deal with on a daily basis. It keeps many people from living the life they so desperately desire. This fear is what keeps many people from taking the first step. Often, the fear is unfounded or simply untrue, but we often become attached to this fear and are afraid to live without it.

Kathy felt that fear very clearly in this chapter. She was challenged to open up and actually get uncomfortable, get *real*. She didn't want to, and she had that voice in her head telling her it was a bad idea. The voice sounded like it was trying to protect her, but it was holding her back from her long-term happiness. That voice is based on fear. We have a much smaller voice inside of us, if only we'd take the time to listen to it. The smaller voice tells us to do it, to go for it, to take the leap. The smaller voice quietly reassures us and builds us up. However, too often, the fear-based voice wins out.

The risk of vulnerability is rejection, when another person pushes you away. It is entirely possible, and I hear about it all the time: Divorce, family grudges, and hardened hearts abound. In these situations, I like the Dr. Seuss quote: *"Be who you are and say what you feel, because those who mind don't matter, and those who matter don't mind."* Don't be afraid of who you are. You are beautiful, vibrant, and full of light. Share your light with the world.

You Are a Gift

You have so much to offer this world. You have talents and treasures that need to be shared. I guarantee you have something inside you that is worthy of its own speech, a conversation several hours long about something deep and profound. Your life experiences and your views are unique, and they can change those around you in a positive way if you let them out.

Ask a friend, spouse, pastor, counselor, or even total stranger to help you. Ask if you can share something that is in your heart. Find a time or a place to be open about an issue you have.

For me, my first step to real vulnerability was in counseling. I was able to "get real" with a person who had no personal investment in my life other than to help me through my struggles. Then, that progressed to sharing with a bunch of total strangers in twelve-step groups. Then, I worked up the courage to share with my church group. That gave me the courage to tell my girlfriend of three weeks my life story. I wanted her to know who I really was, so we could either go forward as our true selves or part ways sooner. We are now happily married and enjoying life with our first child.

Too often, I was willing to settle for relationships based on what I thought others wanted. So, I pretended to be a certain way. I did things in an attempt to anticipate what they wanted or were feeling. In doing so, I never got to be my true self, which made every compliment and praise sting. The person whom they loved and celebrated wasn't really me.

You may not see yourself shouting your struggles from the rooftop, but I guarantee you; if you start small and safe, and grow the practice of vulnerability, it will fundamentally change you. I know it has changed me.

Go out and share your light. If you can't think of anyone to share with, I'd be more than happy to listen. My email is andrew@talltrainer.com.

The Three Bears Approach

"It is about making the wisest possible investment of your time and energy in order to operate at our highest point of contribution by doing only what is essential."

– Greg McKeown, *Essentialism: The Disciplined Pursuit of Less*

Not Too Little

"Too little" knowledge means that you don't know how to do it better. In this age, it is a rarity. With most general issues, we have a rough idea of what it will take to get started. Want to lose weight? It will probably involve changing what you eat or reaching out to an expert to get more ideas. This is what Kathy does. She recognizes the need to get additional movement, accountability, and knowledge. She knows enough to make that first decision. She decides to try and start training with someone local who has a well-established reputation.

If you didn't know that being obese or overweight carries a much higher risk of early death, learning that fact may help you to get the motivation you need to do something about it. Blissful ignorance only lasts until your first heart attack. And then, sometimes, it's too late.

For more specific changes, there may need to be another step. If you've been avoiding exercise for a few decades, you may not know what is available in the fitness world. Research will be key. Google it; email people in the know; ask around. All of these actions combined will yield great information.

If you have too little information, you will not know how to take the next step. Doing some searching, reading, watching, and listening will allow you to absorb enough content and ideas to get that first spark. As you gather new information, don't worry about having the complete picture at first. The most important thing is having enough information to take the first step. Just take the first step, then worry about where to go after that.

Not Too Much

There is a flip-side to learning. If you know "too much", it can actually create "analysis paralysis". This means that you've taken in so much information, reviews, testimonials, and stories that you can't process it all. You become confused and overwhelmed, which quickly leads to disengagement and inaction. You force yourself into doing nothing because you are afraid of making the wrong choice.

This is extremely common when it comes to health and weight loss. The sheer volume of information that gets put out to the general public is impressive, and much of it is contradictory. We think, "A high fat diet is good, but fatty foods have lots of calories. Running is a great way to burn calories, but I've also heard it might be bad for my knees. Strength training is good for muscle building and protecting my bones, but high-intensity interval training is supposed to be the most efficient way to work out. What am I supposed to do?"

If you're like most people, the answer is, "Nothing."

As I worked through the drafts of this book, I took it upon myself to really get to know writing and self-publishing. I read about a dozen books on the topic. At one point, I felt hopeless because not all the ideas and strategies matched up. Worse yet, there was a lot of overlap between each book but also a lot of unique ideas. The sheer number of ways to market the book, set up a writing routine, and bring in other professionals to help, left me perplexed. Which way should I choose? I started feeling depressed and avoided the editing I needed to do.

I had too much information.

Just Right

There is a sweet spot when it comes to learning. You need enough information to be dangerous but not so much that you get overwhelmed. Here is the secret to knowing when you have enough information: You're excited! You see an opportunity, and you are ready to seize it! That means you have enough information to know what to do, but you don't have so much that you've found every single reason *not* to do it.

When you hit the sweet spot, capitalize on it! (We talked about taking action in Part I.) When you feel motivated, fired-up, pumped, excited, or whatever it is you feel when you're ready to do something, *do it!*

GROW YOUR MIND SHRINK YOUR WAIST

Discover Your Habits

"But to change an old habit, you must address an old craving. You have to keep the same cues and rewards as before, and feed the craving by inserting a new routine."

— Charles Duhigg, *The Power of Habit: Why We Do What We Do in Life and Business*

Do you sympathize with Kathy? Maybe you've been snubbed for a promotion, or you have forgotten to do something again and again, or you have fallen into the same pattern day after day. Here are a few statistics that may shake you up: Over 40% of our decisions each day are based on habit. Each year, 50% of Americans attempt to change their lifestyle around the start of the new year. Only 8% of them are successful.

Habits are powerful. They shape us into who we are. In his book, *The Compound Effect*, Darren Hardy talks about how our small, seemingly insignificant, daily decisions will come to define our legacy. Sleep through your alarm every day? Skip workouts? Taste-test your cooking before dinner? Doing any of these things once is not going to destroy you. Over a lifetime, these small issues can have enormous consequences.

Even your small habits matter. They all have the potential to bring you towards the bright and glorious future you envision for yourself. They also may set you up to repeat the nightmare scenarios you've been living in.

Let's take a look at a few of Kathy's habits from back in Chapter One:

- Shopping on autopilot

- Forgetting to water her plant

- No healthy plan for dinner

- Plopping onto the couch after work

Each of these habits carries numerous drawbacks. Each of them consists of three parts. As per Charles Duhigg's book, *The Power of Habit*, the three elements necessary to form a habit are:

1. Cue

2. Routine

3. Reward

Whether good or bad, every habit will have these elements. Let's frame each of these habits as actionable, and we'll explore what they contain and what may be missing.

- Watering the plant.

  o **Cue:** Plant is dying.

  o **Routine:** Getting water from the water cooler.

  o **Reward:** Plant lives!

- Unhealthy dinner.

  o **Cue:** Arriving home from work.

  o **Routine:** Searching for quick and easy food options, finally settling on one or multiple less-than-ideal options.

  o **Reward:** Preserve limited mental and physical energy.

- Plopping onto the couch after work.

  o **Cue:** Being tired after work.

  o **Routine:** Reading magazines and mindlessly eating.

  o **Reward:** Relaxing; not feeling pressured to do anything.

PART II: LEARN

As you can see, even our bad habits have rewards. If you want to break a bad habit, you need to attack at least one of the three essentials:

- **Get rid of the cue.** This is pretty straightforward. The reason Kathy has no recipes or ideas is because she has none prepared. Or if she does, she has no cue to use them. Add one in. Set an alarm to go off when you arrive home, leave your healthy cookbook on the counter, and have your meal plan written on the fridge.

- **Interrupt the routine.** This keeps happening to Kathy as she tries to water her plant. Her routine gets interrupted and is never finished. Now, imagine finding a way to disrupt a *bad* habit.

- **Eliminate the reward.** To curb Kathy's couch habit, she can cut the TV cord or cancel her magazine subscription.

To build a healthy habit, you need to reverse-engineer all three steps. Be sure that your habit has a strong, immediate reward. If it does not, it will not last. Just look at a gym on January 1st vs. January 31st. On the 1st, everyone is packed in like sardines, and there is a wait to try and do anything. By the 31st, most of the newbies have faded, and the gym is at a more tolerable capacity.

Action Step: Identify three negative habits that are holding you back, and three positive habits you'd like to implement. Go through the above exercise. Identify the cue, routine, and reward. Find ways to disrupt the bad habits and build the good habits. Once you've fleshed out all six habits, pick one to eliminate and one to implement, and then, aggressively pursue them. Right now, you have motivation and energy. In a few weeks, you may not. Set yourself up with a reward if you can make it to 30 days sticking with the new habit and eliminating the old habit. (I like to bribe myself with either spending money or a massage!)

Go to www.GrowYourMindBook.com to get a head start on breaking through some of your bad habits with the 10 Day Jumpstart Course. I'll also give you my favorite books and podcasts. I've kept them out of this book as they are certainly open to change, and will definitely need to be updated as time goes on.

Best Ways to Learn

"All I have learned, I have learned from books."
– Abraham Lincoln

I poked a little fun at some current diet fads in Chapter Three. If you have seen success using one of these methods and are willing to stick with it for the rest of your life, I want you to do what makes your heart sing. I have found that the more extreme a solution sounds, the more unlikely it is that people will stick with it for the long-term. Your results are as permanent as the changes you're willing to stick with.

Conversations like the one Susan, Penny, and Cynthia were engaged in can get very confusing for those who are new to these practices. The amount of noise in the weight-loss industry continues to grow as more people look for a quick fix. We're tackling the long-term in this book. By changing our mind and adjusting our perspective, we're setting up our lives to filter down the noise into what is most effective and relevant for us.

It's no coincidence that Kathy ended up in a library at the start of her journey. She needed something to move into the next stage of her development. In the book she found, there was the analogy of the closed door. Obstacles in your path are like locked doors, and it will take a key to open it. That "key" may come in a few different forms.

I believe that there are three keys to growth which will open any door you come across: Action, learning, and purpose. They all play off each other, and we need to cycle between them continuously as we come across new challenges and opportunities. The end of Part I is a perfect example of these three elements coming together to give Kathy direction and a way to continue her story.

A book fell onto Kathy's head. For many of us, this may not literally happen, but often, something like this *does* jump out and hit us right when we need it: The flyer that came to Kathy's home; seeing the library as she was searching for safety. There are examples I'm sure you can think of in your own life. These obvious moments are usually only clear in hindsight. In the moment, they often seem like obstacles, failures, or extra noise.

An opportunity fell onto Kathy in the form of a book. She chose to take action by reading it. As she read it, she started learning more about herself and how to get out of the situation she was in. She learned enough to find a purpose. She was able to ask the right "WHY" question, and she had her purpose.

Right now, Kathy has a simple purpose: To find Bill. As this story develops, we'll see that this purpose will not be enough to sustain and energize her. She'll need to dig deeper.

In his book, *The 7 Habits of Highly Effective People*, Stephen Covey discusses the concept of sharpening the saw and chopping down trees. He links saw-sharpening to learning. As you learn, your saw gets sharper, and your ability to cut down trees improves. If all you ever do is sharpen your saw, you won't be a very good lumberjack. You need to take action and cut down trees, as well. There is a ratio of education to learning that works best for each individual. What I've found is that the sooner I can take action on my learning, the more trees I can chop down.

There is a third element that I have been discussing, and that is to know "WHY". This is what will energize you. A lumberjack with a sharp saw cutting down trees for a bad reason or no reason at all will tire quicker. If you want to sustain your energy and continue to drop trees, purpose will keep your motivation high.

Learning is an essential step on your journey. You must already believe this, because you are reading this book. You think that by learning something new, you can gain a new perspective and ideas, or make a connection that will get you past your pain-point. Pain-points cause discomfort, and we seek to remedy them. Pain comes in many forms: Physical, emotional, relational, and spiritual. Something about this book appealed to you as a solution to your pain. It offered a glimpse of a brighter future, free of that pain.

The bad news is that there is more pain in your future (sorry!). You will have to keep learning, taking action, and fleshing out your "WHY" to get through that pain. As your journey of growth continues, here are a few of my favorite ways to learn, in no particular order. Try to incorporate these into your life as much as you can.

Read Books

I do this in a variety of ways. My favorite is Audible, an Amazon company. It has audiobooks. I have a lot of "dead" time in my life, and I'm sure you do, too. Anytime I'm in the car, working out alone, doing boring chores, or engaging in other, typically mindless activity, I have some free mental space. I use it to "double-dip". This is when I get something done that needs doing, *and* I upskill myself. I learn something that I can apply to a different area of my life.

My second favorite way to read is on my Kindle book reader. I can bring a library with me wherever I go. I've even got the Kindle app for my phone so that if I have "dead" time in a waiting room, or I'm tempted to waste time on social media, I have a quick way to get a few minutes of reading in instead.

Listen to Podcasts

There are a lot of podcasts out there covering almost any subject you could be interested in. Podcasts are like a direct link to a creative and inspirational mind. Often, they are a little more unfiltered and less stuffy than books or articles. Podcasts are a great way to take in information that may not yet be published or widely shared. Podcasts can be much more engaging and dynamic, as compared with other mediums. There may be multiple speakers or a variety of topics and ideas covered.

My all-time favorite podcast is "Hardcore History" by Dan Carlin and his team. I'm a huge fan of story (as you can probably tell), and Dan does an incredible job of tying the stories of history together in ways that make sense and are memorable. He was one of my inspirations for this book.

Find Experts

If you want to lose weight, find a personal trainer. If you want to repair a relationship or recover from trauma (whether new or old), a counselor may be a good choice. If you struggle with knowing what or how to eat, a nutritionist might be right up your alley. Seeing an expert in person will usually cost a pretty penny, but I've found that the value I've gotten in my life has usually been far more than what I paid for. If it isn't, find a better expert! Doing this in-person is a great way to go, but we live in an amazing age of information, and you can access experts from anywhere in many different ways. Skype, YouTube, Facebook Live, Instagram, and Twitter are just a few ways to interact with experts if you can't get to one in person.

Take a course or training. This combines many of the above examples: You'll have an expert on hand; there may be some reading involved; and you may get some hands-on experience. This is another of my favorite ways to learn, because I'm immersed in the subject, and I can learn with others, which usually makes it less expensive. Auditing classes, attending fitness expos, conventions, or educational conferences, joining organizations or clubs, and attending speaking events can all be great ways to learn more. I find that I'm most motivated for change after events like these.

Watch Vlogs and Read Blogs

A wealth of information is right at your fingertips. On the internet, there are articles and videos about almost any topic imaginable. Bloggers have some great tips and support to give, especially about niche problems. If you like the theme of this book, check out our blog over at:

https://www.talltrainer.com/blog

As you continue reading, I recommend paying special attention to the chapters that give you strong feelings, whether positive or negative. These may be the chapters that need a deeper dive. I also encourage you to check out the books that have inspired me, and the extra resources I've included in this book.

PART II: LEARN

Action Step: Pick one of these mediums to continue your learning. If you are feeling really inspired to hire a personal trainer after reading this book, then go do that. If you really want to take a cooking class to improve your meals at home, go for it! One of the crucial mistakes that Kathy made at the start of the book was waiting to call the expert. "I'll get to it tomorrow" really means "never". Instead of waiting for something to fall on your head again, do it now! It'll take less time than you think. Download the Audible app, find and follow a podcast, and contact the expert. You never know when life will jump in to derail your plans…

Lightbulb Moments

With new information and some reflection on things that happened previously, Kathy comes up with a plan. This "lightbulb" feeling is not anything unique or special. It doesn't happen because of a whimsical accident. You can cultivate lightbulb moments as often as you need them in your life. You'll find that, as you apply these steps, the lightbulbs will keep going off, often when you least expect it!

This feeling can be addictive. It feels like an endorphin rush. You reach a new level of understanding and viewing the world. The most important thing about a lightbulb moment is what happens next. What you *do* with that idea or inspiration is the only thing that will matter in a year, five years, or on your deathbed.

I remember taking marketing classes in college, and in one of them, we had to come up with a new product to bring to market. We chose the smartwatch (as did a few other groups). We put together a few ideas and presented it to the class. I guarantee this happened in every marketing class at every college. Yet, almost none of those who "came up with the idea" are working on that type of product today.

What you do with your newfound knowledge is vital. Use that burst of excitement and energy to get started, and then, let momentum help push you through the tough bits. When things are at their hardest, you'll need clarity of purpose to power through. And you *will* have hard times. Expect them. Embrace them. Because that is how you grow.

Creativity, progress, innovation, and motivation all stem from the same root: Growth! If you want to achieve more or get to a new place in life, you'll first need to grow as a person.

PART III
PURPOSE

CHAPTER 9
Mission Disaster

*K*evin and Michelle went ahead of the rest of the group. As the most experienced members of the expedition team, they scouted out the area ahead. Kathy had a lot of respect for the husband and wife team. They had originally been clients of Angela's. They had been so successful at changing their lives that they wanted to join Angela and help her any way they could. They were a great team and made excellent leaders. They had faced hardship of their own and were trying to find their daughter.

Kathy missed her own children. They were safe, but Kathy wasn't sure how long that was going to last.

"Kathy!" Tammy whispered urgently.

Kathy snapped to attention and looked ahead of them.

Kevin was in the second-floor window, giving the go-ahead sign.

Kathy signaled for the rest of the group to proceed. Mary went first, with her husband, John, close behind. Tammy was next. Kathy took up the rear. They didn't move in military formation – quite the opposite. They shambled slowly, almost aimlessly. Their movements betrayed no purpose or liveliness. When they got to the front door of the two-story home, they slipped inside.

Kevin and Michelle already had the cupboards open and were loading their duffel bags with any edibles they could find in the house. They took care to avoid windows, and when they needed to move past one, they would amble slowly by it, avoiding any show of purpose. That was what the trolls keyed in on – purpose, direction.

Kathy reached into a cupboard to grab the cans there. She noticed that her arm looked lean and lithe. The back of her arm especially surprised her. It looked like it belonged to someone else. The feeling of having jiggly, lunch-lady arms was gone. The muscle underneath held firm. Kathy had once joked that she should get an American flag tattooed on the back of her arm, so it could wave in the wind. That seemed so long ago.

She had only been with Angela for a little over two months, but she had never felt better. She missed her husband and children dearly, but her mind was in a better place. Kathy felt like she was actually living, instead of just going through the motions.

PART III: PURPOSE

The training and discipline that Angela helped foster was paying dividends. Kathy felt it all through her body. Strength, endurance, and power. She could keep up with the others on expeditions and was one of the fastest among them over longer distances.

The group finished grabbing the essentials from the bathroom and kitchen and made hand signals showing they were ready to move out.

They gathered near the front door and quietly slipped outside. There was one more house to check. It was the last house on the block before the manufacturing plant where Bill worked.

Kathy let herself hope they'd see him. It was a long shot, but she hoped he was still himself.

The group approached the house cautiously. They had come across trolls in this area before. Kevin tested the front door. It was locked. Michelle signaled to head to the back entrance instead.

That door was locked, too. They began searching under rocks and mats to find an emergency key. Kathy started searching in the side yard under the bushes, near the fence. They didn't want to break any doors or windows, as that was likely to attract unwanted attention.

Kathy crawled towards a lawn ornament near the chain-link fence that separated the yard from the factory grounds. As Kathy reached for the rock, her gaze fell through the links into the factory window beyond. She saw the figure of a man. As he turned, Kathy caught a glimpse of his face.

It was Bill. She was sure of it.

Without thinking, Kathy crawled up to the fence and followed it until she found a section that she could squeeze through. There must have been a dog that lived at the house, because the spot had been repaired multiple times. Right now, Kathy was thankful it was bent out of shape.

Kathy had not taken her eyes off the window since she saw Bill. She needed to confirm it was him. After getting past the fence, she quickly moved through the gap between the factory and the fence.

The room beyond the window was dark. All Kathy could see were the few places illuminated by the sunlight. She placed her hand on the window and watched the glass fog up around it.

Kathy looked back across the field to the house. It was so much farther than she had originally thought.

PART III: PURPOSE

Could I really have seen my husband from that distance? Kathy began to doubt herself.

Motion in the far corner of the room caught Kathy's eye. From the shadows emerged a figure. He was tall, and Kathy recognized the hair on his head. His shape was the same, but different. It was Bill, but not the Bill she knew.

He walked to the window and stood across from her. His face was fully revealed by the light. Kathy lifted her hand to her mouth as she gasped. His face was contorted. The proportions were wrong. He had turned.

Kathy's stomach dropped to the floor. She felt cold all over.

Even Bill.

"Did you get a haircut?" Bill said. The sound of his voice was muffled by the window.

Kathy was taken aback.

He smirked and followed up his query. "No, it's not the hair. You're on some fad diet again. I don't know why you bother with these silly weight-loss programs. They don't change who you really are." He leaned into the window and tilted his head down, so Kathy could see his bloodshot eyes. "I *know* who you really are. In another week, you'll slowly fall off your exercise plan, and it will fade into oblivion, just like every other time. You just aren't a finisher, Kathy."

Kathy staggered back from the window, her face wet with tears. The cold wind seemed to turn them to ice on her cheeks.

As she turned to run to back to the house, she could hear rhythmic pounding on the glass as Bill tried to push his way through.

"You'll never be good enough!" he bellowed.

Kathy ran.

As she reached the fence, she heard the glass shatter. The fence had been pushed out to allow an easy exit from the house. Kathy sat down and pushed her legs through. When she got to her torso, the fence caught on her jacket. She struggled mightily to get it untangled.

Looking behind her, she could see Bill, followed by a horde of other factory workers. Their posture indicated they were up to no good.

Several strong hands grabbed Kathy's ankles and pulled her through.

PART III: PURPOSE

Kathy was thankful to see Kevin, Michelle, Mary, and John, staring back at her.

"Looks like we're in trouble now," John said.

The group quickly left the factory behind.

The morning faded into afternoon as they worked their way down the block. They had two close calls with trolls. Despite the risks, they pushed to a second, then a third block away. They were able to find two more people: Brenda and Tammy.

As they started back down the block, Kathy noticed all the extra people were slowing them down. It looked like Angela noticed it, too. She tried to quicken the pace. It was risky. If they were caught now, it was a long way back to the restaurant.

Angela was leading them back now. It was getting too close to nightfall to try any more houses.

As they meandered back, some of the new group members were getting nervous. They started trying to move closer to the front. They looked too focused. If they were spotted by a troll, they'd be in trouble for sure.

"You're fakers!" a female voice cut through the air. "Why do you bother trying? All of you are worthless!"

GROW YOUR MIND SHRINK YOUR WAIST

Angela yelled, "Run!"

They all broke into a full sprint, some faster than others.

The troll was visible now. She was in hot pursuit.

"Turn here! It's a shortcut!" the troll yelled from the rear of the group.

Kathy looked down the side street as they ran past. It was crawling with trolls. They heard the commotion and joined the pursuit.

Kathy's lungs were on fire. The air stabbed her lungs like icicles dipped in hot sauce. Her throat was raw, and her nose felt frozen. And still, she pushed forward.

They were within a block of the plaza that held the gym and the restaurant. Angela was the first to reach the edge of the block. She turned around and yelled back, "C'mon! You've got this! Finish strong!"

Kathy was exhausted. After a full week of pushing herself in the workouts, she felt like he had nothing left. They rounded the last house, and the sign on the side of the building came into view: *"There is Hope."* Kathy rallied the last of her strength and pushed for the restaurant.

PART III: PURPOSE

Michelle, Angela, and John were the first ones in the door. As Mary, Brenda, and Tammy arrived at the same time, there was a jam in the doorway. Kathy reached the group and dared to look behind her.

Angela's encouragement echoed through the parking lot. The troll rounded the corner of the house.

"You're almost there!"

The troll saw the sign. Angela's words washed over her. It looked like she had been hit by a brick wall. The troll came to a dead stop.

Kevin was behind Kathy now, pushing her into the open door.

Kathy stole one final glance under Kevin's arm.

The figure standing in the parking lot was not a troll anymore. Kathy saw clarity in her eyes.

The rest of the trolls were moments away.

Kathy saw the woman whisper, "Help."

The door slammed shut.

CHAPTER 10
Action Plan

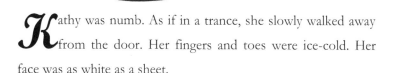

*K*athy was numb. As if in a trance, she slowly walked away from the door. Her fingers and toes were ice-cold. Her face was as white as a sheet.

"What happened out there, Kathy?" Angela asked.

Kathy stared at the ground and answered in a monotone voice, "I found him."

Everyone knew whom she meant. They had all shared so much together, they knew each other's stories. Each person had taken the time to share and get real with the group. It had really helped build the team dynamic and lift each person's individual burden. Somehow, it just helped when other people knew about your troubles.

But right now, Kathy didn't want anything to do with the team.

"You almost got us caught out there!" Mary rumbled as her face turned beet-red.

"Running off like that put us all at risk, Kathy," Michelle said. "We want to help you, but we can't help unless you ask."

Kathy was still shaken. With a stone face and sad eyes, she said, "I can't believe the things he said to me…"

"What happened to your husband is not your fault," Angela said. "He's not himself. Everything he said may sound true, but it's not. He knows you very well; he can hit your deepest, darkest places, but that doesn't mean he's right. You are a child of light; you have so much to give this world. Don't let his words cut you down."

Kathy nodded her head halfheartedly. "I need some time," she said.

Several in the group nodded. The rest had their heads downcast and brows furrowed. The mood was heavy.

Kathy went into the side room and closed the door. She walked toward her meager pile of possessions that were stacked neatly near the opposite wall. When she reached her things, she leaned her back into the wall and slowly slid to the ground. Exhausted, she closed her eyes for a moment.

Kathy awoke, still feeling drained. She was disoriented.

PART III: PURPOSE

What time is it? What day is it?

Kathy flipped open her phone, expecting a full twelve hours to have gone by. As she looked at the time, she became more confused. It had only been a half-hour.

Kathy shook her head as she remembered what had happened that day.

She had put so much hope into rescuing her husband. But he wasn't himself anymore.

Kathy was still alone in the room. She reached for a power bar and tried to replay her meeting with her husband and their hasty retreat. She thought back on all the challenges she had gone through. She recalled the negative ladies at the library, the sweat she had poured into training her body, and the many near-catastrophic encounters with the trolls.

She settled on one memory that still made her palms sweat when she thought about it. As she and the group were running from one of the trolls, she had caught a glimpse of her as they turned a corner and ducked into a building. The woman had stopped chasing them and was staring at her hands. As Kathy rounded the corner, she remembered locking eyes with the woman and sharing a look of confusion and realization.

She had brushed that memory aside, because she hadn't thought it was real. Now, the more she thought about it, the more the puzzle pieces started to align.

What if the plague that was afflicting everyone was based on perspective and attitude?

The trolls had held her down when she was moving purposefully, and the more she fought them, the harder they clamped on. It was as if they hated her purpose. Nothing but hate and discouragement poured from their mouths. It was an unending barrage that sucked the life out of her.

That had to be it. They were people who had no mission, no reason to do anything. They just wanted everyone to be like them – to shut others down and avoid the pain of change. The three library ladies came to mind. They had been "normal" at first. They had spouted nothing but negativity and did nothing to change their situation. And they'd all changed that same night.

Now, she had to find a way to get all the trolls to wake up. She thought back to the glimpse of the woman she had seen. Her eyes had been so alert, no longer cloudy like they had been only moments earlier. Her face had regained its color and was no longer contorted. She had woken up.

PART III: PURPOSE

As Kathy thought back to her time at the library, a jolt ran through her. She knew what they had to do.

Angela shook her head. "It's too risky; we can't know for sure that it will work," Angela said.

The group was gathered in the main exercise room. Kathy's idea had not been received well.

"If it fails, we'll all be toast. We'll be too far from the gym and too tired to get away," Michelle chimed in.

"This is all hinging on what you think you saw when we were pumped full of adrenaline after running full-tilt for almost a mile. I don't see how we can go through with this," John said.

Kathy looked down for a moment. She couldn't let it go. Too much was at stake. She had come too far and lost too much to have it be for nothing. They had to try it.

"Remember when you found me?" Kathy replied.

Kevin and Michelle nodded their heads solemnly.

"I was totally spent. I had nothing left to fight them off. I had given up. As soon as I resigned myself to that feeling, they left. It was like their only mission was to get me to quit. Having succeeded, they left and went on their sad and depressing way.

"They want to destroy all things good and exciting. The day before this whole mess happened, I was on the verge of falling into a deeper spiral of depression. I hated what my life had turned into. I hated my job. My marriage was dull, and the purpose of my life – my two children – had moved over 1,000 miles away and didn't want much of my help anymore. I thought I was as low as I could get.

"Then, I saw one of your darn fliers, Angela," Kathy said.

Several in the group smirked. Angela's fliers were known to get people riled up. She had received complaints about them in the past because they were too real. People were sometimes offended by their bluntness. But she kept sending them, because they got people to take action.

"I vowed to myself that I was going to make a call the next morning. I'm convinced that's why I woke up still in control of myself that day. Because I had a new purpose. It was only the thread of a purpose, and my head and heart weren't totally in it yet. But it was enough to get me through the morning.

"Then, I saw firsthand how it has all been negativity-based. Everything that is good and exciting has either reversed or kept the plague at bay. That is the key. We need to spread *positivity*. These things are walking sad-sacks. They need help. And we can help them. We have exactly what they need. It isn't about our survival anymore. We need to change them. We need to take this positivity that we've grown here and put it out into the world.

"I've given up on myself before, but I'm not going to give up on all of them. I'm not giving up on my husband or my kids. They all need what we've got. You said you all wanted to help me. If I'm going to do this, I need your help."

Angela shook her head again. "We don't have any proof. It's one thing if we knew this disease could be reversed, but it's too big of a gamble. I can't justify the risk."

"I thought so, too," Kathy said. "That's why I want you to meet someone."

Kathy walked to the side room and opened the door.

A woman stepped through the doorway. She was petite with brown hair and had a business suit on. Her eyes and face were clear and focused. She stood tall and spoke with confidence.

"My name is Karen," she started. "I feel like the last few months have been a bad dream. I can remember the day of the storm, and how the lightning came down, and my outlook became cemented. Before then, I was lonely and miserable. I worked for an accounting firm that treated everyone like cattle. I hated hearing the alarm clock go off each morning, because it meant that I had to go back. After that fateful day, I wanted to share my misery. It was like that lighting strike turned me from passively miserable to actively miserable. So, I spent my time trying to bring others down. I didn't realize what had happened to me. I didn't understand that I had become a troll."

The room was silent as she paused.

"And then, I saw all of you. I saw how hard you were working, and I couldn't stand it. It was like your success was a bad reflection on me. I know it sounds crazy. All you were doing was running home, but I took deep and personal offense to that."

The group was all intently focused on her, nodding slightly. Angela leaned back in her chair. All eyes moved to her.

"I'm in," Angela said. She stood up and embraced Kathy. The rest of the group hollered and piled into the moving mass of excitement.

CHAPTER 11
Race Day

The cool air of winter was fading into the crisp brightness of spring. It was still cold. But today, it felt warmer. Today was the day they were attempting the impossible. Kathy had convinced the group to give her idea a fair try. Now, she had her doubts.

Kathy and the rest of the group had surveyed the town and found where most of the trolls had congregated. The fastest runners of the group were in position, scattered throughout town. Michelle, Kevin, and Angela had snuck out early that morning and set up near the largest concentrations of trolls. The others in the group were crouched and waiting near the library.

Kathy stood out in the middle of Main Street, half a block from the finish line. She reached into her jacket. Raising a pop gun into the air and pulling a bullhorn to her mouth, she yelled, "RUNNERS, READY!"

Her voice echoed down the quiet street.

"SET!"

Figures started moving in her direction.

"GO!"

POW! The pop gun let off a loud blast. That was the signal for her runners to go.

Kathy ran back to the rest of the group, sensing the motion all around her as trolls emerged from driveways, doorways, and around corners.

They had estimated it would take their closest runners about ten minutes to reach them.

Kathy held her breath as she looked at her phone. She started the timer.

Everything hinged on Kathy's hunch. As she arrived back with the main contingent, she could sense the nerves of those around her.

Several tense minutes went by. Kathy anxiously checked her watch. She promptly forgot what it said and had to check it again.

PART III: PURPOSE

The others could tell she was nervous. They started fidgeting more, too.

They could hear the growing murmur before they saw anyone. At the nine-minute mark, Kathy could see a runner come around one of the side streets to her right. After a few moments, another runner arrived to her left. Then, another. Each of the runners had a trail of trolls running after them. Angela was at the head of one of the masses of runners. It looked like she was being chased.

They all converged on Main Street at about the same time. Angela was slightly behind the other two runners. All of them had what Kathy hoped were people hot on their heels.

Kathy signaled for her team to step out and into action. Karen handed out drums, tambourines, and other noisemakers. Brenda spray-painted a line across the width of the street. John and Mary pulled out a tall banner on poles and fixed it into position. It read: *"Congratulations! You made it!"*

They all took up positions on the edge of the road and began making an awful ruckus. Many of them had cardboard signs. The others played all sorts of noisemaking devices. They were all cheering for the trolls.

Michelle was the first runner from the group to make it. Kevin was close behind. As each of them crossed the finish line, the groups that had been following them fused into one as the funnel-shaped road brought everyone together.

Then came Angela, followed closely by a bellowing herd of trolls. Angela had her earbuds in, and it was clear that she couldn't hear a thing the trolls were saying, as her smile had never been bigger. Angela looked winded but enthusiastic. She shot Kathy a warm smile and a wink.

With less than one hundred yards to go, the worst happened. Angela tripped while running past a curb and fell, sprawled out on the ground.

For a brief moment, the group stopped their chanting and cheering, and held their breath.

The trolls chasing Angela were closer than Kathy was. There must have been hundreds of them. They came bearing down on Angela. Kathy imagined them all swarming her and shutting her down.

The next troll behind Angela closed in. Twenty feet. Ten feet. Then, he was on her. He grabbed a hold of her arm. Kathy couldn't bear to look.

A cheer went up from her crew. She turned back to look. Angela was on her feet, being pulled towards the finish line by the other runner – a human runner. The runner who, until that morning, had been a troll. Kathy couldn't believe it. She shrieked and started yelling encouragement through the bullhorn.

Angela and the other runners started crossing the finish line at a rapid pace. The team quickly spread out and started looping medals over necks and handing out t-shirts that read: *"Running for Readers"*. Kathy had hoped the library shirts and gear would be the final touch in getting those people rehabilitated.

Each of the runners that crossed the line looked bewildered and confused. But they were smiling, and so was Kathy. She said a quick prayer of gratitude and joined in as more people crossed the line.

Whooping and hollering, she could see the wave of change go through the chasing trolls. As they approached the finish line, their features changed. She started recognizing some of the faces. She saw her neighbor, Ben. One of Bill's coworkers, Kevin, transformed as he crossed the finish line.

As the former trolls got their bearings, they began to chant and cheer as more and more trolls crossed the finish line. As they crossed, the curse faded. Each twisted face turned into an ear-to-ear smile.

The positivity and enthusiasm was contagious. It worked!

In the chaos of the post-race celebration, Kathy came face-to-face with Bill. He smiled at her. His eyes were clear and bright. He was back. They held each other for a long moment and kissed. It was a moment of pure joy. Kathy never thought she'd have him back again. It was a beautiful moment.

The surging of the crowd pushed them into the library parking lot, then began to disperse.

"How are the kids? Are they okay?" Bill asked, sadness in his eyes.

"They're safe for now," Kathy said. "Now that I have you, I'm not letting you out of my sight again." Kathy's look made it clear that she was only *slightly* joking.

Kathy reached forward to embrace her husband again, partly for comfort and partly just to confirm that he was still with her. As she held him tightly, she glanced over his shoulder. Kathy's mouth dropped at the sight in front of her.

The parking lot next to the library was slightly higher than the rest of the area around them. It gave a decent vantage point to see most of the downtown area. The streets were packed with people. Kathy had thought that most of the town had turned into trolls. During the race, it had seemed like an endless horde of them.

That horde paled in comparison to what Kathy saw now. The streets leading into Main Street were crowded as survivors poured out of their hiding places.

Angela walked up to Kathy and Bill.

"It's wild to think that the tyranny of the minority had so much power over all of us," she said.

Kathy and Bill nodded somberly.

"All it takes is one person willing to stand up and take a chance. Thank you for being that person, Kathy."

Kathy blushed and accepted the compliment.

The crowd grew tighter, and Angela slipped away in the mass of bodies. The morning sunlight caught Angela just right, and Kathy thought she could see wings. Kathy blinked, and they were gone.

CHAPTER 12
Full Circle

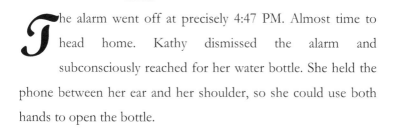

The alarm went off at precisely 4:47 PM. Almost time to head home. Kathy dismissed the alarm and subconsciously reached for her water bottle. She held the phone between her ear and her shoulder, so she could use both hands to open the bottle.

"Thanks for all the information there, Ted. Are there any other concerns about our progress in Morocco?"

"No, that just about does it!" Ted replied. His voice sounded tinny through the phone.

"Perfect. Let's plan on having another update on Thursday, same time," Kathy said.

After finishing their conversation, Kathy poured water from the open bottle onto her ficus. In the two years since the beginning of "The Great Troll Resurgence", the ficus had seen massive improvement. It used to fit nicely on top of her desk. Now, she had to keep it next to her, as it was over a foot tall and had started blocking her view from across the desk.

She smiled, thinking about how that plant mirrored much of the growth she had experienced since "Troll Day," the first day of The Great Troll Resurgence. Many had taken to calling it T-Day for short. The afterglow of the successful race in her hometown had been short-lived. There were episodes occurring all over the United States and many other nations.

With the encouragement of her husband and her new friends, she held a 5K in the neighboring town. Then they did another and another. They formed a non-profit organization and began spreading their ideas and opening new chapters across the globe. Kathy was thrust into the role of CEO. It was very uncomfortable for her at first, but she took to focusing on helping others and continuing to grow as a person.

The effective use of positive energy was contagious. It kept the trolls at bay and saved millions from the same fate. As a matter of fact, the "Run for Purpose 5K" had become the largest charitable organization in the world, in terms of volunteer hours. People were on board with the mission.

Kathy looked back at the phone on her desk and smiled again. She had just hung up with her former boss, Ted McGovern. He had survived T-Day but had not been able to leave his home until after the 5K had cleaned up the town. He had been one of the first volunteers to help in the subsequent races. He was also one of her hardest workers, and her most reliable manager of setting up new operations. He was in charge of the African division of the company.

Kathy stood up from her desk and walked to the door, which was perennially open. She strode through it and was greeted by her secretary and personal assistant, Michelle.

"Don't forget; you have dinner tonight with your kids," Michelle said with a smile. "Based on the meal plan you laid out for the week, I ordered some extra spinach and sweet potatoes. You've got some extra mouths to feed!"

Kathy returned the smile. "I'm thankful they are able to stay in town for the night before they head back out in morning."

The kids had been stranded at their college after the epidemic had spread to them. Kathy had been able to talk them through how to organize the race, and the type of encouragement that worked best. Since then, both Jacob and Hannah had been a part of the mission to spread positivity throughout the world.

"Can you have the extra ingredients dropped off, so I can get home sooner?" Kathy said. "I don't want to miss a minute with them!"

"Absolutely!" Michelle replied. "Isn't it amazing what technology can do these days?"

Kathy was thankful for the modern convenience. It may have cost a bit extra, but the benefits in cases like this made the added cost seem cheap by comparison. Time with family was precious, indeed.

"I also wanted to remind you of your workout with Angela tomorrow."

"How could I forget that?" Kathy said as she rubbed her still-sore glutes. "I've been remembering that last workout all day!" They both chuckled. It had been a tough one that morning.

"I'll see you tomorrow!" Kathy said. "If you're all set on your end, you can pack things up and head on home, too."

"I've got a couple of loose ends to tie up here, and then, I'll be on my way," Michelle said.

As Kathy walked through the rest of the office, she was greeted by many warm smiles and waves as her other employees packed up their desks. She counted herself as truly lucky to be able to make such an impact on the world.

When Kathy started her car, it automatically picked up where she had left off in her audiobook.

> "If you aren't failing, you are stagnant, and change is coming for you, whether you are prepared or not. The title of this book is Action Required because that is the most important step to take. But if it's all you ever do, you will never achieve your true goal. You need two other ingredients: You must know WHY, beyond all shadows of doubt, and so deeply that when you have a choice of an action to take, it will be an obvious decision. The other step in this repetitive process is to LEARN. This is where that failure benefits you. Without learning, your failures will bring you crashing back to the unstable ground of life."

It was her favorite book, *Necessary Action Required*. She had downloaded the audio version and listened to it at least once a month during her commute. Kathy estimated that she had gotten through at least ten other books per year just during her driving time. And she had definitely needed it. As the need grew for something to combat the troll epidemic, Kathy had to grow her company, as well.

Many methods had worked at combating the trolls, but by far, the most economically effective method had been setting up the race environment. The energy, positivity, physical exertion, and positive atmosphere all conspired to turn trolls into productive members of society once again.

Kathy pulled into her driveway and noticed that her husband had beat her home. He loved and fully supported the work she was doing, but he had come to enjoy the camaraderie at his old job. He changed his frame of mind, and that made all the difference. Their marriage had grown closer, and their mutual support had ushered them into a second dating life. They truly enjoyed their time alone together now. It was like they were newly married again.

Kathy walked up the front steps and opened the door to the kitchen. She could see her husband preparing dinner. Kathy turned around to close the door and take off her shoes. Before she could turn back around, her husband held her in a tight embrace.

"Welcome home, darling!" he said as he wrapped his arms around her and took a deep breath in her long hair. "How was your day?"

"Oh, you know…" Kathy let the statement hang in the air for a moment. "Just trying to save the world."

They both laughed, because it was certainly true.

They set about preparing the food. When Jacob and Hannah arrived, it was a truly merry scene. The house smelled of sweet potatoes, salad, and barbecued chicken. The summer sun dipped below the horizon late in the day, and it wasn't long until yawns began to pepper the conversation as much laughter.

The family said their goodnights and got ready for bed. Jacob's room had been turned into a guest bedroom. He made himself at home. Hannah, a bit younger, hadn't had her room converted yet, so she felt nostalgic as she looked at the posters of her favorite bands from high school that littered the walls.

Kathy and Bill got into bed together and turned off the lights.

"I'm thankful this troll epidemic happened," Kathy said, seemingly out of the blue.

In the darkened room, Kathy could sense Bill cocking his head sideways. "What makes you say that?"

"Well, I was just looking back over the day. And the past couple of years." She paused for a moment to fully gather her thoughts.

"I realized that our lives are completely different – and for the better – because of that experience."

Kathy could sense Bill nodding. She continued, "I never would have thought in a million years that we would be where we are today. Looking back at how things used to be, I never could have imagined being here today. It makes me wonder; what's next?"

Bill chuckled. "Yeah, you might be running for president someday!" His tone indicated that he thought that was quite the longshot.

Kathy threw a throw pillow at him at point-blank range. It bounced off of him and landed softly next to the bed.

"I could, you know!" she said.

"I know," Bill said, his voice suddenly very serious. "I know you could, honey, and you'd be great at it."

Kathy felt her heart swell. He always knew how to say the right thing.

"I can't help but feel like things are too good right now," Kathy said as her mind brought forth all the possible ways that her new life could come crashing down.

PART III: PURPOSE

"I think we are in a good season right now," Bill said, his voice smooth and confident. "I believe there will be more challenges to come, and we are still in the midst of a struggle. There are plenty of parts of the world that still need our help. Your work is changing lives, *saving* lives."

Kathy felt more reassured. Bill continued, "Our work here will never be done. I think that's some of the trouble we ran into a couple of years back. We thought our jobs were done. We got stale and stagnant. There's always more to do, and more ways to learn and grow."

With that, they held each other tightly. Whether it was a way to hold onto the present or protect the moment from the uncertain future, Kathy couldn't be sure.

As Kathy drifted off to sleep, she wondered what her workout was going to be in the morning.

Purpose Lessons

Purpose Separates "Good" from "Great"

"Good is the enemy of great. And that is one of the key reasons why we have so little that becomes great. We don't have great schools, principally because we have good schools. We don't have great government, principally because we have good government. Few people attain great lives, in large part because it is just so easy to settle for a good life."

— Jim Collins, Good to Great: Why Some Companies Make the Leap... and Others Don't

Kathy came to a closed door in Chapter 9. Her husband hit on the very thoughts Kathy had already been subconsciously feeding herself. The result was devastating. What she did next is a defining trait of those who have a growth mindset.

After all her efforts, she hit a major obstacle. Her husband wanted no part of her help, and he was certainly no help to her. With all that emotional turmoil, Kathy had a choice. Here, the path between a growth mindset and a fixed mindset splits. A fixed-mindset person takes the defeat as a sign that it was not a worthy goal to pursue after all. That person thinks the pain and suffering have all been for naught. The pain that person feels is paralyzing, and they wallow in it, unwilling to move on from it. That pain comes to define them. It is a mark, a scarlet letter, a brand burned into them, announcing their failure to the world.

Thankfully, Kathy has grown into a growth mindset. She understands that a setback is only temporary. She sees that there is an opportunity to get better, and work through the obstacle. She begins to apply the three-step process we've been exploring in this book.

First, she absorbs and processes what just happened. I would encourage you to do the same. Set time aside to dive fully into the emotions that may be whirling around inside you. Failure to do so is like trapping a storm in a glass bottle. You'll have to keep releasing pressure from the lid to keep it from exploding. That pressure release tends to involve bad habits, addictive coping mechanisms, and a sure path to frustration.

By processing her feelings, Kathy is able to move on to the start of a solution. She recognizes that some of her trouble came from her *purpose*. It turns out that trying to rescue a person who doesn't want to be rescued is a losing battle. She understands she needs to focus on something different and more productive. However, she still wants to be proactive in the process, so she's not waiting for things to "sort themselves out".

PART III: PURPOSE

By working through emotions and challenges, you will set yourself apart. Because you are willing to take the time and energy to invest in yourself, you are saying to the world that you are better than "good enough". By figuring things out and taking action, you move into the realm of greatness.

Build Your Tribe

"A tribe is a group of people connected to one another, connected to a leader, and connected to an idea. For millions of years, human beings have been part of one tribe or another. A group needs only two things to be a tribe: a shared interest and a way to communicate."
— Seth Godin, *Tribes: We Need You to Lead Us*

The people you are surrounded by will have a profound effect on the way you act and behave. We become like those we spend the most time with. Who are the top five people you spend time with? Chances are, your income, mindset, and attitude aren't all that different from theirs.

Kathy made the choice to stick around and get to know this group. She chose to integrate, instead of going it alone. By teaming up and pooling their resources, her chances of survival and success improved dramatically. Humankind has worked this way for millennia. It is in our souls and DNA. We function best with other people. They say, "If you want to go fast, go alone. If you want to go far, go together." Groups offer support, both physical and emotional. Within the group, there is protection and security. There is a sense of belonging that helps us feel safe and allows us to let our guards down.

Your approach to exercise and eating will probably encompass a lot of your "tribe". Your beliefs and habits in these areas will help create your body shape. I recommend jumping right in. If something feels right, go for it. As a trainer, here is what I focus on when it comes to clients: Safety, results, and fun. I think a great exercise class needs all these elements. All these will tie back into your overall purpose for pursuing exercise. There are many reasons to go after it: Health, longevity, feeling good, competition, camaraderie, self-care, recovery, freely expressing yourself, testing your limits, etc. Each reason will steer you towards a different type of tribe. Often, it takes both action and learning to see which things are truly the most important to you. Research, experiment, and reflect on what you want to get out of the time you spend exercising and changing your attitude towards food.

PART III: PURPOSE

The 3 Essential Elements of Your Fitness Tribe

The most important aspect of a fitness facility needs to be safety, both physical and emotional. Many people are terrified of a gym environment, so the instructor needs to be the guardian of the environment. Physical safety is often related to the exercises being performed. Much of this comes through training and experience. Look for a trainer who has been in their field for multiple years. Check for certifications; make sure that it took more than a weekend retreat to become qualified for what they do. Qualifications are only half the battle. Make sure your trainer has a personality that can motivate and inspire you. Most gyms and studios will let you test or view their programs to see whether they match what you're looking for. I highly recommend doing this. It will allow you to get a quick glimpse into the trainer's everyday work. If you like what you see, jump right in!

The next important thing is results. This is what will keep you going for the long-term. If results are the least important, then eventually, you'll become frustrated and move on. Look for testimonials or a "Transformation Wall" at the gym you're looking into. They should have lots of results, and plenty of raving fans to talk to you about all their benefits. If they don't, consider moving on.

However, if results are #1 on the importance list, there can be trouble, as well. It can become very performance-based, with risky and short-term thinking winning the day. That means increased risk of injury, crash diets, and negative peer pressure. These elements leave people hurt, dissatisfied, and oftentimes, in worse shape than they were when they started!

Now, here's the element most people look for first when they go to the gym: Fun! It is an essential element in an exercise program. If the first two are taken care of, then fun will probably happen naturally. Look for a personality that fits well with yours. If your instructor is super dry and sarcastic, and you appreciate warm goofiness, you may not have much fun. Stage presence is critical here. If your instructor comes in with low energy and does not inspire you to be better, laugh, and enjoy yourself, you'll be ready to move on before your contract is up.

Take a look at the people in the room, their general fitness levels, age, and disposition. You'll start to become like these people if you hang out with them long enough. Are they the type of people you aspire to be like? If not, that's a sign that this may not be the right place for you.

Action Step: Here are the things I recommend looking for as you continue your personal growth journey: A group of people to exercise with and a nutrition plan that resonates with you, both now *and* two weeks from now, when life gets harder.

I recommend exercise groups for one major reason: People miss you when you're gone. You can get the same effect with a personal trainer. Accountability is *massively* important. Without it, you will fade away from your routine because staying home on the couch is much easier. Find a place where you feel connected, alive, energized, and fulfilled. These places used to be rare, but fitness is becoming more ingrained in our culture as a useful necessity, so quality options are becoming more widely available.

What to Look for in a Trainer

Kathy found an amazing trainer who also happened to be her fairy godmother. Your trainer may not have wings, but I believe there are many people out there who can help you unlock your true potential. You have greatness caged inside you; you need to find the right person to help unlock it.

I want to help you find the best quality trainer in your area. Here are a few things your trainer should have and be able to do:

- **Professional:** If it looks like they do training as a hobby, their level of training and expertise may be marginal. Look for someone with full-time training experience, either current or in the past. Like any craft, trainers get better over time.

- **Able to modify:** If you have injuries, limitations, or anything else that will make certain activities or exercises dangerous for you, your trainer needs to be capable of meeting that need.

- **Personality match:** Make sure your personality, sense of humor, and energy levels come close to matching. If the trainer is super high-energy and off-the-wall with enthusiasm, you will need to be the type of person who thrives on that. If you're more of a wallflower, then you may seek out a more grounded personality. However, remember that sometimes, choosing an instructor or class that pushes the boundaries of what you are used to may help you grow.

- **Practice what they preach:** Your trainer should be in good condition. They need to have a body and lifestyle that matches what they are coaching others to achieve. I love the saying: "Leader of one, leader of many. If you can't lead one, you can't lead any."

PART III: PURPOSE

Nutrition: Think Long-Term

When it comes to nutrition, everyone has an opinion. Here's mine: Your results are only as permanent as the changes you're willing to stick with. If you are looking into a nutrition plan, make sure you can definitively say that you want to continue it forever. How many times have you started a diet and gotten great results? Are those results still around? Most likely not, or this book would not have jumped out at you. So, how many diets have you tried that didn't work?

There are so many named diets out there: Atkins, keto, paleo, vegan, vegetarian, etc. I think we don't have enough. There's only a few thousand options out there. We need to think bigger – in the hundreds of millions. I'd like to see a diet named after every man, woman, and child in America. It's time for you to go on the "[Your Name Here] Diet". It's named after you. I'm on the "Andrew Diet". Mine has chicken wings in it, and cookies that my wife bakes occasionally. It's also got lots of vegetables, plenty of water, and great protein sources. My point here is that there are so many differences between our bodies without even factoring in our preferences. There are food sensitivities, allergies, intolerances, and things you just plain don't like. You need to experiment with what works for you.

GROW YOUR MIND SHRINK YOUR WAIST

I heard a great quote from an interview done by Tim Ferris. He was interviewing a YouTube celebrity, Shay Carl, and asking him about his weight-loss transformation. The Shay said "I thought to myself, 'The secrets to life are hidden behind the word cliché.' So any time you hear something that you think is a cliché, my tip to you is to perk your ears up and listen more carefully."

Look for the tried and true; it'll be more likely to stick for life.

Accountability

Lastly, your tribe will provide you with accountability. It will keep you true to your purpose. These people will push you to grow in a particular direction. That's why determining which direction you want to grow in is essential. It is the foundation you will build your habits and lifestyle on.

If you love competition, then find a place that uses it to sharpen its members. If large groups scare you, find someone to work with one-on-one or in small groups. Wherever you end up working out, make sure you will have a reason to roll out of bed when the weather is bad or you just don't feel up to it. Those days come more often than most people like to admit.

PART III: PURPOSE

Put Your Earbuds In

"What other people think about you has nothing to do with you and everything to do with them."
— Jen Sincero, *You Are a Badass: How to Stop Doubting Your Greatness and Start Living an Awesome Life*

The runners had earbuds in as they were being chased by the horde of trolls. It wasn't just because that's what runners tend to do. It also represents something bigger.

Not everyone in your life is going to like the changes you are making. As a matter of fact, many people will be defensive and downright hostile about what you're doing. Too often, we listen to those voices – the trolls – because they are repeating words we've already told ourselves. They bring up some of our biggest fears and deepest wounds.

As you find your purpose, something will start to change in you. That purpose will expand to the point where it encompasses all of you. You go from doing to *being*. You go from doing healthy things, to *being* healthy. That process takes time and consistency. That purpose, that state of being, gives you focus and clarity. You can see your goal. You can imagine and feel what it would be like to get there. And you understand there will be habits, thoughts, and even people who will need to fall by the wayside to let your spirit truly roar. As those shackles of your past beliefs fall away, you'll be free to live your truest purpose.

Before all that exciting and deeply fulfilling work happens, though, you're going to have haters. There will be people and situations screaming in your face to stop pursuing these important tasks and the vision you have. It will be uncomfortable and discouraging. You might be tempted to quit. The more you change, the more pushback you'll receive from the universe. It will seem like everyone and everything is conspiring against you to stop you.

This is when you put your earbuds in.

I don't curse much, and this next sentence is the only time I will in this book:

You need to proactively drown out all the crap that is coming at you and stay focused, because your life is too damn important to let other people decide what you do.

Seriously.

I want you to give yourself the level of respect and encouragement you deserve. Cultivate and nurture your own mental thoughts. Block out the haters. And follow the path. It will be winding. It will have cliffs and washouts. It may even disappear at times. But you have to keep going. Your life – your happiest and most fulfilling life – depends on it.

Know "WHY"

"Working hard for something we don't care about is called stress:
Working hard for something we love is called passion."
—Simon Sinek, author of *Start with Why: How Great Leaders Inspire*
Everyone to Take Action

A person with a strong sense of purpose is like a magnet. They inspire, teach, and lead. Their direction is clear, and they aren't led astray by distractions. They pursue what is great and leave behind what is merely good.

Martin Luther King, Jr., Thomas Jefferson, and Steve Jobs exemplify this concept. They were able to shape the world around their mission, their purpose, their "WHY". "WHY" is a big deal. Kathy started exploring that in this last part of the story. She got clarity on why she was pursuing her husband, why she needed to bring him back into her life.

In his bestselling book, *Start with Why*, Simon Sinek details how a strong foundation built upon a well-thought-out "WHY" will shape how a business or person behaves. If you know why you're doing something, your actions will become completely clear.

You'll know where your deficiencies are. You'll know where you need to seek expert help. You'll know how to resist temptation.

This is one of the keys I've found in every person I've trained who has sustained their weight loss and body change. They know deeply why they are doing it. Saying "no" to things has become easy. Getting up early to work out has become natural. Taking the hard road has become essential. It has become a part of them, instead of just something they are doing for a bit.

Your initial "WHY" for pursuing something may change. I started writing this book as a way to grow the business I work in. It took me two and a half months to get halfway through the rough draft. Then I discovered a better "WHY" – I have knowledge and a way of presenting it that I know can help people. This book can change lives and mend hearts. I wrote the second half in less than two weeks.

And then I spent the next five months avoiding it, because I was afraid it wasn't going to be well-received. When I did work on it, I was editing it to death in fits and spurts. After many conversations, I realized the general reception of this book didn't actually matter. What mattered was that it could help *one* person. I hope *you* are that one person. I hope this book can open up new doors for you. I hope this way of thinking can give you deeper purpose, and a system to fall back on when you hit a plateau.

PART III: PURPOSE

Knowing why helps you engage your "elephant," your steam engine, the part of your brain that gets you emotionally turbocharged. You'll have strength and staying power. You'll achieve your dream, and you'll be able to maintain it and grow from there. People who have a poor "WHY" will sometimes achieve the goal they set out for after much hardship and personal sacrifice. And then, they'll start to regress. This is what "yo-yo dieting" is.

Yo-yo dieters are pursuing their goal of losing weight with a bad mindset. If you've gained and lost weight (15+ pounds) multiple times in your life, you fall into this category. Want to break the cycle of dieting and bingeing? The cycle of up and down? The cycle of nearly reaching your goal and watching it slowly come undone?

If there is one thing to learn from this book, it is this: Your mindset influences everything. You need to put yourself into a growth mindset to take control of your life and make real, lasting progress. Your goal of weight loss is only part of the picture.

Your weight only represents your relationship with gravity. That's it. It's just a number. From a sales perspective, that is a feature. A statistic. What really gets you fired-up is the benefit. Being lighter or in better shape will cause something to happen. You'll experience a better life in some way. The features of being lighter are many. You'll need smaller clothes; you'll reduce health risks; you'll put less strain on your joints. The benefits are that you'll feel more confident, and you'll live a longer, more fulfilling life. There are many more features and many more benefits, but the "WHY" is what will really get you motivated.

Not sure how to dig into your "WHY"? Get going on the 10 Day Jumpstart Course at www.GrowYourMindBook.com. I've created a 10 Day email course to get you started on your journey.

Dig Deeper

Every minute of quiet time and self-reflection that you give yourself will multiply its benefits tenfold in your life. It's no surprise that some of the most successful people in any avenue of life are the ones who take time for meditation and prayer. These same people will often keep a journal and reflect on things that went well and things that didn't.

If you're not willing to create time for self-care in this way, you will always feel like you're on the hamster wheel of life. You'll be exhausted and ready to drop, but the wheel will keep spinning. You'll either hold your ground or steadily get worse in every area of your life, unless you dedicate time to making things better. Self-care is how that happens. Give yourself twenty minutes in the morning for some meditation, reading, and journaling. Find things in your life to be thankful for. As you expand this practice, you'll find even more things in life to be thankful for. And things to be thankful for might start finding *you!*

Be a Hero

"Extreme Ownership. Leaders must own everything in their world. There is no one else to blame."
– Jocko Willink, *Extreme Ownership: How U.S. Navy SEALs Lead and Win*

Kathy has changed. You could argue she has made a full transformation. Her approach to eating and exercise has certainly changed, as proven by her leaner physique. Her mindset is different. When she is confronted with obstacles, her reaction used to be defeat. Now, she tries to figure things out. She learns, experiments, and tries to understand the deeper issue. She recognizes that waiting around for change to happen on its own will not work. She takes a stand for what she knows is right. These are all the traits of a leader. She has begun by leading herself.

Leadership helps you just as much as it helps others. As you change and become a better leader of yourself, you will begin to influence others. A leader is not necessarily a formal role. All it takes is a follower to have a leader. If you start having a positive impact on others' lives, you will positively affect them and take on a leadership role. Leadership provides accountability. If you're leading, you're more likely to follow through on expected behaviors. You may learn more about yourself as you help another through a shared struggle.

Being a leader of yourself means that you are willing and able to face the brutal facts of the situation. A leader will see the depth of the problem, no matter how scary or embarrassing it may be, and take action on it.

Kathy is following the growth opportunities she sees in front of her. As one door closes, another one opens. If there is no open door, perhaps there is another way through instead. Your troubles and obstacles will follow a similar path.

Kathy has stepped into her future potential. She has ceased playing the part of spectator. By going after what she feels is right, she has been richly rewarded. She has saved her husband, her town, and herself. She has undertaken a hero's journey. She has found a mentor, a group to keep her motivated and accountable, and a new method for living life going forward.

You are the hero of your own story. You are its central character. You also get to write much of the story. You hold the pen. A few parts will be written for you; there may be tragedy that strikes or an errant coffee spill onto the paper that jeopardizes the rest of the text. As you continue to write more of your story, you may feel that you're not ready, or you're unworthy, or that the thing you seek is not meant for you.

Always remember who is holding the pen. Personally, I believe that *I* am holding the pen, and that the hand of the divine perfectly encapsulates mine as we write my life story together.

AFTERWORD

Kathy has come a long way since the first chapter. Her story was designed to show how a change in mindset can alter the reality you live in. Kathy is still the same person. She's just in better shape, has a more exciting career, and much deeper relationships. This is possible for you, too, and I think it's the reason you picked up this book.

This book is based on many of the practices we use at the studio I work in, Tall Trainer Fitness Systems in Canandaigua, NY. Our program is designed to take someone who has a lot of reservations about exercise and turn them into a confident, capable, and growth-focused exerciser. We call our program "Bootcamp" because it serves the purpose of rapidly integrating a person into a group culture and gets them ready to take on larger tasks. We draw a lot of parallels to military bootcamp – though we've left out the miles of running, and the screaming and cursing. You're welcome.

Military personnel must all go through basic training to continue in the armed forces. They are put through numerous tasks and challenges that build confidence, trust, and a growth mindset.

GROW YOUR MIND SHRINK YOUR WAIST

Those who are falling behind in the early days are pushed and challenged until they reach a level of competence they may not have known they had.

This book is bootcamp for your mind. I hope you have been challenged and pushed in new directions. I hope the ideas in this book have shifted your perspective on health and fitness. I know the keys of Action, Learning, and Purpose can serve you just as well as they have served me. A growth mindset is the most powerful tool you can have. Knowing you can put in the work and reap the reward is truly freeing. It opens up an entire world of possibilities that may have eluded you for a long, long time.

A growth mindset does not always apply universally within the same person. Some people have a growth mindset when it comes to their career, but a fixed mindset when it comes to relationships. In that respect, we see the cliché of the corporate climber who has experienced a divorce or two. A growth mindset is not a guarantee for a happy and successful life. The ideas of happiness and success are completely subjective.

What a growth mindset *can* do is give you the keys to the locked doors in front of you. How you feel after you walk through those doors is up to you. The keys of Action, Purpose, and Learning must be used in an ongoing cycle to fuel your growth.

AFTERWORD

Kathy's story has been one of ups and downs, of successes and failures. By applying a growth mindset, you're signing up for both sides of the coin. You'll learn from your failures and find great personal benefit from your successes. What you'll also find is that both your successes and your failures can be used to help others along, as well.

Go out into the world and share the good word! Hope is not dead. Better health and fitness is possible. If you want the possible to become permanent, all you need to do is continue to grow.

ACKNOWLEDGMENTS

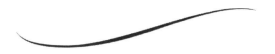

I'd like to give all glory to God in this. Through Him, all things are possible. And through His love and grace, my life has been totally transformed. He has put the people, resources, and ideas into my life that brought change and growth, which inspired me to help others do the same.

I am thankful for all the encouragement I received as I worked on this book. I felt fragile as I created something with great effort, not knowing how it would be viewed. I am eternally grateful to my wife, Samantha, who has pushed me and allowed me to take countless hours to work on this project. She was even relatively enthusiastic about me working on it during our vacation!

Thank you to all the staff at Tall Trainer. A special shout-out to my brother, Jeremy, for supporting me in this process. Sarah, your notes on my rough draft were incredibly helpful and pushed me to get this done. Just seeing that someone enjoyed it was enough to push me to finish this!

To all my clients, both current and former, thank you. It is for you that I wrote this book. I see your struggles. I recognize the pain you go through when it comes to change. This is my attempt to help you. A few of you may recognize pieces of your own story in here. A special thanks to you for being vulnerable and willing to share such tough memories. You helped these characters come to life.

Thank you to my family for listening to my drafts and crazy ideas. I loved our brainstorming sessions.

Mom and Dad, you were the ones who got me to finally pull the trigger on the wild idea of writing a book. I can vividly remember our conversation over dinner at a fancy restaurant. Thank you for always having faith in me and encouraging me to take big leaps.

I need to give a shout-out to one of my mentors, Todd Durkin, for pushing me to be better every day. Thank you for putting together an incredible group of fire-breathing dragons to help change the world. It was during the lead-up to your mentorship event that I was able to get focused and dream up the basis of this book. I'm uncaged now! Watch out!

ACKNOWLEDGEMENTS

I'd also like to thank two teachers who had an outsized impact on my development as a writer. Brian Moore was my high-school language arts teacher, and he took my work seriously. His insights and genuine enjoyment of my writing gave me confidence at a time when I needed it most. Curt Nehring-Bliss was my creative writing professor at the Honors House at Finger Lakes Community College. His courses inspired and challenged me to write in ways that were uncomfortable and helped me grow. Thank you, Mr. Moore and Professor Nehring-Bliss.

Finally, thank you, dear reader. You were the one this book was written for. Not the masses, not the critics, and not even myself. During my toughest moments of self-doubt and crushing insecurity, it was by thinking of only you that I was able to carry on. If this book can help just one person (you!), then it was worth the effort.

ABOUT THE AUTHOR

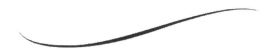

Andrew Biernat is a Certified Personal Trainer, speaker, coach, and newly-minted author. He holds associate's and bachelor's degrees in business administration, as well as the premier certification in the fitness industry, Certified Strength and Conditioning Specialist (CSCS). He leads classes and coaching sessions in his hometown of Canandaigua, NY, at Tall Trainer Fitness Systems, with his brother and company founder, Jeremy Biernat.

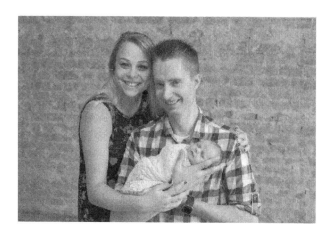

Andrew has been training since 2013 and has helped restore hundreds of bodies and lives to the glory of God.

Andrew is a loving husband to his wife, Samantha Biernat. They were married in September of 2016. In July of 2018, they welcomed their first child, Rosabelle, into the world. The Biernats love the outdoors and spend a lot of time at their family cabin in the southern tier of New York. They also occasionally binge-watch shows on Netflix.

Just for You

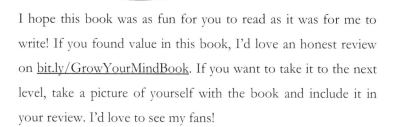

I hope this book was as fun for you to read as it was for me to write! If you found value in this book, I'd love an honest review on bit.ly/GrowYourMindBook. If you want to take it to the next level, take a picture of yourself with the book and include it in your review. I'd love to see my fans!

If you're looking for more ways to grow with me, I encourage you to check out www.GrowYourMindBook.com. You can connect with me there, book me as a speaker, or inquire about coaching. I'm giving away a free 10 Day Jumpstart Course to get you going on your wellness journey. Take some ACTION now, then we'll start LEARNING and finding your PURPOSE for getting healthier.

Made in the USA
San Bernardino, CA
09 November 2018